Written Communication in Family Medicine

Written Communication in Family Medicine

By the Task Force on Professional Communication
Skills of the Society of Teachers of Family Medicine

Edited by

Robert B. Taylor, M.D.
Katharine A. Munning, Ph.D.

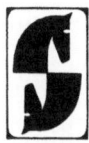

Springer-Verlag
New York Berlin Heidelberg Tokyo

Robert B. Taylor, M.D.
Department of Family Practice
The Oregon Health Sciences University
  School of Medicine
Portland, Oregon 97201
U.S.A.

Katharine A. Munning, Ph.D.
Department of Community and
  Family Medicine
Duke University Medical Center
Durham, North Carolina 27706
U.S.A.

Library of Congress Cataloging in Publication Data
Main entry under title:
Written communication in family medicine.
  Includes index.
  1. Family medicine—Authorship.   2. Medical writing.
I. Taylor, Robert B.   II. Munning, Katharine A. [DNLM:
1. Communication—Methods.   2. Family practice.   WZ 345
W956]
R729.5.G4W75   1984   808'.06661   84-5408

With 6 Figures

© 1984 by Springer-Verlag New York Inc.
Softcover reprint of the hard cover 1st edition 1984

ISBN-13: 978-0-387-90979-0   e-ISBN-13: 978-1-4612-5248-1
DOI: 10.1007/978-1-4612-5248-1

Preface

This work presents the knowledge and skills necessary for successful written communication in family medicine. It is intended for use by teachers of family medicine who, as part of their academic responsibilities, are called upon to produce written documents in a wide variety of areas. The book has also been written to serve as a resource for leaders presenting faculty development activities in various aspects of written communication, including writing for publication, administrative and educational communication, and other topics of interest to academicians.

The Task Force on Professional Communication Skills was formed in 1981 as an initiative of the Board of Directors and the Communications Committee of the Society of Teachers of Family Medicine (STFM). In early meetings, the Task Force defined its goal as improvement of the communication skills—both written and oral—of STFM members. A survey of Task Force members revealed that the greatest challenges lay in the area of written communication skills, although the needs are not confined to medical article and book writing, but extend to the full range of academic communication. The Task Force set as its first task the creation of a monograph on written communication in family medicine.

The work that follows is a joint effort of the Task Force on Professional Communication Skills and a group of selected authors. Robert Taylor has been the project coordinator; Katharine Munning has written the faculty development activities for each topic. The editors wish to thank the authors and the STFM staff members who have worked on this project.

We hope that our fellow STFM members find the following chapters useful.

Contents

Part III   Administrative Communication

Part IV   Educational Communication

Part V   Common Interest Areas

Contributors

Carole J. Bland, Ph.D., Department of Family Practice and Community Health, University of Minnesota Medical School, Minneapolis, Minnesota, U.S.A.

Don W. Bradley, M.D., Duke-Watts Family Medicine Program and Department of Community and Family Medicine, Duke University Medical Center, Durham, North Carolina, U.S.A.

Joan S. Carmichael, Ph.D., Department of Epidemiology and Public Health, University of Miami School of Medicine, Miami, Florida, U.S.A.

Lynn P. Carmichael, M.D., Department of Family Medicine, University of Miami School of Medicine, Miami, Florida, U.S.A.

Thomas E. Crowder, B.D., M.L.S., Division of Graduate Education, Department of Family Medicine, University of Miami School of Medicine, Miami, Florida, U.S.A.

Bruce F. Currie, Ph.D., Sisters of St. Mary Regional Family Practice Residency, Kansas City, Missouri, U.S.A.

E. P. Donatelle, M.D., Department of Family and Community Medicine, University of Kansas School of Medicine-Wichita, Wichita, Kansas, U.S.A.

John J. Frey, M.D., Department of Family Medicine, University of North Carolina School of Medicine, Chapel Hill, North Carolina, U.S.A.

Gay C. Kitson, Ph.D., Department of Family Medicine, Case Western Reserve University School of Medicine, Cleveland, Ohio, U.S.A.

Pamela LaVigne, Department of Family Practice and Community Health, University of Minnesota Medical School, Minneapolis, Minnesota, U.S.A.

Jane Barclay Mandel, Ph.D., Department of Family Practice, Medical College of Wisconsin, Milwaukee, Wisconsin, U.S.A.

Maureen M. Moo-Dodge, M.A., Title III, Minneapolis Community College, Minneapolis, Minnesota, U.S.A.

Katharine A. Munning, Ph.D., Department of Community and Family Medicine, Duke University Medical Center, Durham, North Carolina, U.S.A.

Susan Okie, M.D., Department of Family Medicine, University of Connecticut School of Medicine, Farmington, Connecticut, U.S.A.

Joseph E. Scherger, M.D., Department of Family Practice, University of California-Davis, Davis, California, U.S.A.

Robert B. Taylor, M.D., Department of Family Practice, The Oregon Health Sciences University School of Medicine, Portland, Oregon, U.S.A.

Part I

Writing Skills

Chapter 1

Elements of Composition

John J. Frey

Idea Development

The scribes of ancient Egypt were among the earliest groups of writers. They held a special place in the culture of that time, serving as the conduit for information, both mundane and sacred. Excavation of the cities of artisans who constructed the temples and tombs of the pharoahs has revealed a mixture of letters, prayers, shopping lists, contracts, and general messages among people of the time. The scribes were not, I imagine, writing for readers 3500 years later. However, scholars now use those shopping lists and contracts to understand ancient Egyptians better and, by inference, understand ourselves.

Being a scribe is also a craft. Various individuals in early Egypt could sculpt, draw, sing, or govern. Others had responsibility for developing the craft of writing. Although a difficult occupation, it was one full of pleasures. As one scribe wrote to his son in 1400 B.C. from Deir el Medina in the Valley of the Kings:

There is no office free from supervisors except the scribes. He is the supervisor! The office of scribe is greater than any office. There is nothing like it on earth.

We are the scribes of the late twentieth century. Our literature becomes a time capsule.

Writing is a historical act. The role of written communication has been to document human history; our knowledge of human culture and values exists because someone has written about it.

Biomedical writing has its place in the documentation of the growth of ideas. It represents one view of the world we live in, its truths and its problems. Family medicine as a subset of that world has a particular view. The interdisciplinary nature of family medicine offers a wider range of experience and, consequently, a wider range of writing than most other medical disciplines. For that reason also, what we say will affect more than our own corner of medicine.

Ideas contained in the literature of a discipline reflect the values of that discipline—what is important. Our own assessment of the need to alter those values often determines whether we write something. Finally, writing depends on the relative value we see in doing so for ourselves and for our contemporaries.

Although authors report that the lack of an idea is a major impediment to family physicians writing (Curtis, 1981), most writing fails, not for lack of an idea, but from the authors inability to master the mechanics of writing. We do write every day even if we do not write for journals. However, the relationship of writing in patients' charts to writing for a biomedical journal audience is analogous to the relationship between singing in the shower and performing a solo with the local symphony. Either transition is made only through work, practice, and pain. This monograph will discuss problems with style, format, and protocol, and make suggestions that will help the writer do a better and more successful job of written communication. A monograph will not generate ideas. We must do that for ourselves.

The great American physician-writer William Carlos Williams repeatedly stated, "No ideas but in things." Williams' work illustrates that phrase through its range of stories and poetry drawn from his experience as a family doctor. Most of our ideas come from the "things" of our lives as physicians and educators in constant contact with others.

Reading

One invaluable source of ideas is reading. We become involved with our discipline through the things we read. Journals provide ideas which we use to change how or what we teach, or the way we care for patients. In addition, reading creates connections between our own experience and what others have written. Those connections help develop new ideas— different ways of seeing—that can be used or studied. The generalist nature of family medicine as an academic discipline is both exhilarating and intimidating. A narrow subspecialty field has well-defined limits with a narrow range of subjects and style. Family medicine has very few limits, opening up all of experience to scrutiny and discussion. For example, a recent issue of *Family Medicine* contained articles on hyperkinetic children, microcounseling, cross-cultural medicine, patient education, medical student teaching, and epidemiologic research. The levels of discourse in a generalist discipline range from the cellular to the cultural.

Careful reading increases research skills through increased familiarity with methods and research design. Reading the literature also provides a sense of language, important to those who also want to become better writers.

Reading alerts us to the likely audience for our writing. The "house style" of a particular journal is not clear from the guidelines on the "Instructions to Authors" page. The comparison of the British and the American literature usually yields the lament that, although Americans can write, the British write better. Although this is often attributed to an almost mystical gift of language, there is little mystery involved beyond the attention paid to writing, particularly stylistically correct writing, in the British educational system. Thus the "look" of articles in the *British Medical Journal* and the *Lancet* is different from their counterparts in the United States. There is no difference in the instructions to authors, or the format for reporting research. Nevertheless, there is a "style" that is apparent and must be considered if one chooses to write for British journals.

For example, the following statements both address the subject of hemorrhoids:

> Hemorrhoids are varicosities of the hemorrhoidal veins. Those located above the dentate line and involving the middle hemorrhoidal plexus are termed internal hemorrhoids. They are covered by a mucous membrane and are insensitive to pain or pressure. Thus they can be incised, frozen, or squeezed without inflicting pain. External hemorrhoids, on the other hand, are located below the dentate line. They have a squamous epithelial covering, involve the inferior hemorrhoidal plexus, and are quite sensitive. Patients may have internal or external hemorrhoids, and some individuals may have both; those who have both types are said to have mixed hemorrhoids.

> Few who reach middle age can claim never to have had any symptoms related to the anus. Thompson has shown elegantly, if not originally, that what many regard as piles are normal vascular cushions. We all have them, and they are as natural as the vascular cushions at the upper end of the alimentary tract that we call lips. We are prepared to accept a wide variety of lips: thin lips, pouting lips, petulant lips, wet lips, and even hot lips. Similarly, variations in the vascular cushions at the anus should possibly be regarded as signs of character rather than disease.

The first is from a journal containing review articles on various topics—the second is an editorial from a widely read international journal. The style of each would be unacceptable for the other. Reading a range of publications will provide writers with a sense of the research and writing style appropriate for submitting manuscripts to a a particular journal.

Journals also reflect what editors and reviewers consider to be "important" or relevant in a discipline. The decision to accept an article is partly scholarly and partly marketing. While the field of family medicine has few limits on ideas, various journals within the field clearly represent appropriate biases—usually determined by the audience that the editor or publisher sees for the journal. The author's task is to find a "home" for an idea by reading the available literature and deciding where the ideas best reside. Doing this well avoids unnecessary rejections and the pain involved in those rejections.

Medical writing has changed considerably in the past century. Prior to the formation of organized medical journals in the seventeenth century, communication among scholars took place through books. Early books such as Harvey's work on circulation were the cumulative expression of an individual's work in a scientific field. The pattern of journals in this century has been to report periodic developments in a field over many years. Occasional "state of knowledge" texts, such as Cecil's early text of 1927, were meant to summarize a work in a general or specialized field. The rapid expansion of content in any one field often makes large texts become quickly "out of date" requiring 3- to 5-year revisions in an attempt to remain current.

Journal articles have changed in other ways. Articles in journals from the early part of this century were generally descriptive in nature. Since the curative aspect of medicine lay primarily with surgeons, many articles were collections of cases, often by practicing physicians, suggesting one surgical approach or another. Research was prospective or descriptive, emphasizing the natural history of disease. Most journals were regional and, perhaps because of this, most authors did not use large numbers of citations to relate their work to a body of knowledge.

Since that time, the type of research has changed as has the structure of reporting research. Fletcher and Fletcher (1979) reported that over the past 30 years, research in general medical journals has become more cross-sectional in nature and prospective research is marked by shorter follow-up periods. In addition, more articles are now written by multiple authors. In the early days, articles were written in a more discursive, exhortive style representing an individual's thoughts and opinions. The trend to multiple authorship added to the obfuscation that characterizes much of today's medical language. Reliance on jargon and medical clichés reflects the anemic status of "doctor-speak" in the larger context of the English language.

There are differences of opinion, of course. Day has said:

Some of my old-fashioned colleagues think that scientific papers should be literature, that the style and flair of an author should be clearly evident and that variations in style encourage the interest of the reader. I disagree. I think scientists should indeed be interested in reading literature and perhaps even in writing literature, but the communication of research results is a more prosaic procedure. (Day, 1979)

Northrop Frye (1981), on the other hand, while pointing out the different uses of language in science, philosophy, and poetry, argues for a greater interaction of those uses, recognizing their interdependence and the need for a common social purpose. Whichever emphasis an author chooses, his/her language should emphasize clarity and simplicity in the communication of the idea and purpose of his/her work.

Organizing the Idea: Preliminary Steps

The first step after developing an idea of interest is to *write it down*. If the original thought is unclear, one can waste much time and effort elaborating on it. The initial stage in designing a research project is to write down the question or thesis; it is an approach that holds true for any idea that might be the basis for a piece of writing. It starts the process of defining terms and weighing the value of an idea.

A more elaborate statement or abstract is the traditional method of summarizing or condensing a piece of work into its essential elements. While it may make sense to write an abstract toward the end of writing a paper, a working abstract can serve as a guidepost for the process of writing. Continually referring to it while writing will bring the author back to his/her original purpose and avoid the tendency to wander off on to favorite themes or tangential points of "interest." Continually asking, "is what I am saying now related to my original idea?" is a useful technique for keeping to the point.

The next step is *choosing the best format* for fully developing an idea. The range of formats is extensive: research article, review article, commentary, short report or communication, letter to the editor, and others. Again, familiarity with a number of journals helps find the appropriate "fit" between an idea and the method of expressing it.

The format for reporting research is familiar and reproducible. Many articles and texts go into greater or lesser detail about systematically reporting research results, which is not to say the process is easy. Lack of experience in reporting research is one reason many faculty members lack confidence in writing. After struggling with articles published in major medical journals, one appreciates the difficulty that even "experienced" writers have writing clearly. This is particularly discouraging when one realizes that most articles have been through multiple rewrites and have been edited by copy editors.

The third step is *developing an appropriate outline*. Outlines can be quite detailed or very broad. The outline should serve the writer's purpose rather than follow some standardized form, and will make a writer actually set pen (or typewriter key) to paper. An outline may be inhibitory or unnecessary in some circumstances. A letter to the editor, a short essay, a brief report of a new idea, or variation on a problem might be impeded by a detailed outline. Personal journals, pocket binders, or scraps of paper with thoughts scribbled on them have served many writers as sources for organizing thoughts. The trick is to find what works.

Principles of Composition

Composition is often confused with style and should not be. An understanding of the essentials of playing notes enables the musician to develop an individual style or way of playing. Similarly, composition is the fundamental element of writing. Sitting down to write expecting great prose and lucid statements to emerge from one's fingertips would be comparable to picking up a saxophone, blowing into the mouthpiece, wiggling the fingers, and wondering why what comes out does not sound like Charlie Parker. One may even have the talent, but it still takes practice.

Two references that anyone seriously wanting to write must have are: *The Elements of Style* by William Strunk, Jr., and E. B. White (1979), which has been recommended to most of us since junior high school, and *Why Not Say It Clearly?* by Lester King (1978). Strunk and White is the essential text of American English style and usage. Lester King's wonderfully well-written book approaches the language of medical writing head on and shows us how to control it.

Recommendations from both books fall into general categories: Verbosity, Passivity, Pomposity, and Humility.

Verbosity

Perhaps the most common problem in any piece of writing is the presence of too many words. All authors struggle with saying what they want to say and frequently end up saying it too elaborately. Most journals give general guidelines for the number of pages that are acceptable for scholarly articles. This does not mean an author should strive to submit the maximum number of pages permitted. Not only do long articles frequently contain repetitive sentences and paragraphs but also length may interfere with the reader's understanding the piece. One needs to say what is necessary and no more. Each paragraph should contain one or two points; more than that deserves another paragraph.

A concise and tightly written paper will receive a more favorable review than a longer, more rambling one. The content of most journals is determined by the decision of a peer review panel. Shorter papers, if they contain the essentials of the work and its implications, will be read more thoroughly than longer ones, since reviewers get as tired reading long papers as anyone else.

After the first draft, one should go through the paper paragraph by paragraph questioning whether a particular thought deserves a paragraph or can be combined into another paragraph and still be clear. Look at the paper first at the level of paragraphs, then sentences, then particular words or phrases. Most manuscripts can be reduced by 25% after this process without losing meaning or style. Look on a first draft as a "padded" piece of writing wherein lies the real meaning of the article.

A good example of a sentence which should be eliminated is: "Family medicine is a new (emerging, developing, in-its-second-decade, has come a long way, etc., etc.) academic discipline...." If an audience has never heard of family medicine (limited at this point in history to Stone Age members of tribes in New Guinea, although they probably have another name for it), then it might be important to include such a sentence. However, it is gratuitous if the article is intended for a family medicine readership.

Prepositions

King mentions what he calls the preposition ratio. If a sentence contains prepositions at a rate of greater than one preposition for every four words, then the sentence should be examined for ways to eliminate prepositions. Although no rule is absolute, this one helps examine sentence structure in a systematic way.

Specific ways to drop prepositions from writing are:

Drop an entire prepositional phrase. Favorite objects for such deletion are "in order to," "in terms of," "for the purpose of," which often grace medical writing.

Convert the prepositional phrase to an adverb: "by surgery" becomes "surgically."

Convert to active voice: "The study was to terminate when 300 patients were entered" becomes "The study terminated after 300 patients were entered."

This last maneuver also meets another objective by more forcefully expressing an idea in the active voice.

Modifiers

Adjectives and adverbs can enrich language if chosen correctly. Good writers are said to agonize over choosing the exact adjective which will make the phrase more compatible with his/her intent. Many sentences contain strings of adjectives and adverbs which remind one of reading a menu which describes a hamburger as a "juicy quarter pound of choice beef."

Generally, two does not say it more clearly (or better) than one.

"The resistance *and* criticism of some of our colleagues..."

"I was intrigued *and* pleased with the editorial..."

Whenever the word "and" appears, a general principle is to examine the words or phrases on either side to determine whether both are necessary or whether one can be eliminated without losing the meaning of the sentence.

Noun-modifiers provide the source of most jargon. A noun-modifier is a noun that modifies another noun.

"patient management decisions"

"residency-trained family practice graduates"

"frequency data"

"drug abuse treatment evaluation"

Alexander Haig's legacy as Secretary of State may be the gerrymandered modifiers and verbs that amused those who listened to him. Medical writing is no less a treasure house of neologisms. "Prioritizing," "input/output," "meshing," and "feedback" all originated with computers, just as "MIRPing" a patient sprung from "medspeak."

Passivity

Most articles and books about writing—medical or otherwise—bemoan the continuing use of passive voice. Editors of medical journals will encourage a movement away from the use of passive voice, then, in the same issue, publish articles dense with "was performed," "was observed," "is needed," "are summarized," and so on. Passive voice is appropriate in many situations. However, its persistent use is unnecessary, particularly when using the active voice would make a stronger statement.

As an exercise, try putting all sentences in a paragraph in active voice. Such an exercise will produce a different sense of what one is saying. Another exercise is to underline all *is* and *was* phrases in a paragraph, then systematically question whether those phrases best serve the purpose of the statement or can be altered to active voice.

Similarly, encountering "there is" or "there was" should make the writer consider restructuring the phrase in a more active voice or deleting it.

Putting statements in positive form is a corollary to the principle of emphasizing active voice. When possible, say what is intended in a positive rather than negative manner. For example:

A rotating internship may no longer be considered sufficient evidence for eligibility to practice medicine

becomes

A rotating internship may be insufficient evidence for eligibility to practice medicine.

This change eliminates both the passive voice and the weaker negative form of the statement.

Pomposity

Editors ask reviewers to state whether an author's conclusions are justified by the findings presented. Authors, therefore, should take pains to make claims only which emerge from the data. The excitement of completing a research project and reporting results often spills over into the statements used to discuss the conclusions. Avoid words and phrases such as:

major	meaningful	it is clear
critical	central	it is obvious
important	valuable	it is reasonable to assume
significant	essential	it is interesting to note

The reader will decide for him/herself whether findings of a research project are "important" or "reasonable," modifiers which generally can be dropped altogether. "Significant" is a word with statistical meaning in the case of research.

The use of phrases such as "is made explicit by the preceding discussion," "as noted above," "as previously stated," and the like, often seems more condescending than helpful. If the author feels compelled to remind the reader, presumably affected by short-term memory loss, of some point made on the page before, then the author should question the clarity of his/her writing or shorten the article considerably.

Humility

Humility refers to the practice of avoiding strong or positive statements through the use of qualifiers such as:

perhaps	potentially
likely	may
seemingly	might
possibly	

Discussion of methodological problems or biases is a requirement for an author reporting research findings. A good scientist acknowledges the limitations of a study as well as the degree to which findings may not be generalized. However, readers often find a paragraph or two of apologies, followed by a discussion liberally sprinkled with qualifiers that diminish the conclusions. A final sentence that says "larger studies of this type are required before further conclusions can be drawn" hedges all bets.

The overall impact of qualifiers is to weaken the paper, particularly in the discussion section, which is the second most read section of an article after the abstract. The balance between overstating and understating conclusions is difficult to maintain. Careful writers will say what can be said clearly, directly, and as positively stated as the data will support.

Other Helpful Hints

The four principles of Verbosity, Passivity, Pomposity, and Humility do not cover many commonly occurring errors of grammar and syntax. Sentences often lack parallel structure, modifiers are separated from the noun or verb to which they belong, and pronouns and prepositional phrases are vague or confusing. Run-on sentences plague writers who are anxious to "tell-all." General overwriting is the product of uncontrolled enthusiasm coupled with an unwillingness to pay attention to basic rules of composition. Abraham Bergman once said: "When you raise your guns to fire, select your target carefully. A broadside just makes a lot of noise."

Revision and Editing

Once the first draft of an article has been completed, an author can begin the revising process immediately or put the article aside for a few days to let the ideas settle. This is also a good time to have a critically constructive friend or colleague review the manuscript for general comments or specific criticism. An author's ego is less fragile at this stage than it would be after a "final" draft. Specific requests from the author regarding length, clarity, or general effectiveness of the article help reviewers focus their criticisms. Make sure that reviewers meet your needs as an author. Similarly, when you are asked to edit someone else's paper, ask that person what, if anything, he or she would like you to emphasize in your review.

Liberal editing and revision make for better writing and thicker skin. A systematic approach emphasizing principles of composition and grammar is the least painful way to learn to revise. We must be literary critics as well as critics of bad science, criticizing how we write as carefully as what we write about. We should become our own best critics.

Style

While there are rules of grammar and general principles of composition, there are no rules for style. E. B. White (1979) says:

> In this final chapter we approach style in its broadest meaning: Style in the sense of what is distinguished and distinguishing. Here we leave solid ground.

Style is the author's individual voice and involves a matter of preference as well as a sense of "rightness."

Style depends on the audience. For instance, in the standard medical presentation style:

> Mr. Snowdrop is a 68-year-old unemployed white male, chronic bronchitic, with a past history of trigeminal neuralgia preceded seven years earlier by a Bell's palsy on the ipsilaterial side.

F. J. A. Huygen in *Family Medicine: The Medical Life History of Families*, (1982) said:

> Mr. Snowdrop was a fisherman living in an old brick house on the riverside, with two very old lime trees in front, pruned in the shape of two enormous candelabras. When the town was bombarded in 1943, he was there and witnessed how many were killed in his immediate vicinity. It was then that he stopped working and that his illness started: a tic douloureux of the left facial nerve due to a trigeminal neuralgia. Seven years before he had had a Bell's paralysis on the same side with ensuing long-lasting disability. He also had chronic bronchitis.

Both are grammatically and structurally correct and represent styles that, like different languages, serve different purposes.

We write for others to read, not for them to read aloud. The written word has a different sound than the spoken word. A flavor, a nuance, a change of timing from internal to external, for example, makes a screenplay substantially different from the novel from which it was adapted, even if the words are the same in both.

Our published work, whatever form it takes, should represent something that reads well. Developing an individual style requires reading and analyzing other writers. Our style, like our lives, is a combination of our innate sense of language coupled with what we have learned through experience.

Faculty Development Activities

(1) As presented in this chapter, we develop ideas about our discipline from our readings. List the names of the reading materials (i.e., books, journals, newspapers) that you read to develop your ideas about family medicine. Review your list with other members of your faculty. These lists will provide good ideas for additions to your personal or program library.

(2) Develop a short reading list for yourself for the next week or month which focuses on a topic you are particularly interested in such as geriatrics, family dynamics, patient education, etc. After you have completed your reading, make a list of ideas you would like to read about that topic—what questions/concerns do you still have about the topic?

(3) Take an idea from the above list and write it as a clear, concise sentence(s); outline the content that would be necessary to adequately communicate your idea. You are on your way to adding to the literature in family medicine.

(4) Find an article or two that you have enjoyed reading and have commonly used as a reference. Review these articles for the following principles of composition:

   (a) Verbosity

      Does each paragraph contain one or two points?

      Do sentences contain prepositions at a rate no greater than one preposition for every four words?

      When "and" appears, examine words on either side to determine if both are necessary.

   (b) Passivity

      Determine if written in passive voice. If so, change a sentence or two to the active voice.

      Note negative statements. Write these in the positive form.

   (c) Pomposity

      Does the author make claims substantiated by the data?

      Are the following avoided:

      major   meaningful
      essential   valuable
      significant   crucial
      important   it is clear
      it is obvious

   (d) Humility

      Does the author apologize for or diminish conclusions?

      Are the following avoided:

      perhaps   potentially
      likely   may
      seemingly   might
      possibly   could

References

Bjork RE. The careful writer and the sound of words. J Community Health 1981;6:275–81.

Cummins RO. Learning to write: Can books help? J Med Educ 1981;56:128–32.

Curtis P, Nagel D, Ilderton, P. Writing skills for family medicine faculty members. Fam Med 1981;13:8–10.

Day RA. How to write and publish a scientific paper. Philadelphia: ISI Press, 1979.

Fletcher RH, Fletcher SW. Clinical research in general medicine journals. N Engl J
    Med 1979;301:180–4.
Frye N. The bridge of language. Science 1981;212:127–32.
Huygen FJA. Family medicine: The medical life history of families. New York:
    Brunner/Mazel, 1982.
King L. Why not say it clearly: A guide to scientific writing. Boston: Little, Brown
    and Co., 1978.
Strunk W, White EB. The elements of style. New York: MacMillan, 1979.

Chapter 2

On Writing: Getting Started, Getting Stuck, and Getting Finished

Gay C. Kitson

If you think you are alone in having problems writing, be reassured. You are not. Getting started, getting stuck, and getting finished are common problems not only for "part-time" writers like us but also for those whose livelihood is writing. Russell Baker reports that after 20 years of doing so, starting to write his thrice weekly *New York Times* column is still hard (Berkov, 1982). And, Ernest Hemingway rewrote the last page of *Farewell to Arms* 39 times before he was satisfied with it (Plimpton, 1963).

Trouble in translating thoughts to paper can occur at a number of points. Here the concern is not with grammar, format, or sentence structure but on what other writers have found aided them when they were actually faced with the task of composing something. Although the focus of this chapter is writing for publication, the same concerns and issues occur in writing grant applications, memos, reports, or letters.

Getting Started

Be it known: "No dodger is more artful than the reluctant writer" (Tichy, 1966:17). Why is it that staring at an empty sheet of paper and actually being forced to start to write is so daunting? The answer in part relates to the process itself and in part to excuses potential writers use to avoid starting at all. In this section, we shall examine both of these issues.

The Creative Process

Although some authors speak with varying degrees of enthusiasm about the pleasure they derive from discovering new insights and sharing their thoughts with others, virtually everyone who discusses the subject also says that writing is "troublesome," full of "difficulties," "tiring," "lonely," and "frustrating," (see, for example, Tichy, 1966; Elbow, 1973; King, 1978). No wonder people are reluctant to begin!

Luthe's (1976:5) definition of creativity hints at some of the reasons why writing is difficult. He defines creativity as "the ability and facility to actually produce, make, or express something that, at least in part, originated from oneself." Much of the difficulty in doing this is in allowing ourselves the freedom to stop being self-conscious, let the mind roam freely, look at facts in a new way, express thoughts openly, and be spontaneous, imaginative, flexible, and tolerant of ambiguities (Maslow, 1967; Stein, 1974). To allow ourselves to lose control in this way can be frightening. In addition, we may not be sure we want to know what is lurking around in our minds, fear that it will be too revealing, lack confidence in our judgments, or dislike criticism from others.

Often, too, we expect too much from our first efforts. Those who write on creativity in general or writing as a specific form of creativity discuss each as a *process*. It involves (1) *preparation*, gathering data; (2) *incubation*, letting the mind work on this information on nonconscious levels; (3) *illumination*, developing the idea; and (4) *verification*, revising and polishing the idea (Wallas, 1926; see also Tichy, 1966).

To enhance the likelihood of being creative requires a safe external and internal environment that is comfortable and relaxing in order to allow these processes to occur. Writers describe a process of becoming detached from or oblivious to the surroundings or that a narrowing of consciousness occurs. As Abraham Maslow (1967:49) notes, in these circumstances, the influence of other people lessens so that behavior is less affected by them. In this way "we can devote ourselves, self-forgetfully, to the problem."

To describe writing in this way does not mean that we have to wait for inspiration or despair of ever having anything interesting to say. As with learning to do a physical exam, play tennis, or cook, writing is a *set of skills* that we can learn how to do better by watching how others do it, collecting pointers from colleagues about better ways to do it, and by practicing. One method of learning some of the ropes and obtaining some support and guidance initially is to write with someone else who has already published and is willing to serve as a guide. He or she may be willing to share unanalyzed data, an interest they have not had time to follow-up, or an interest similar to yours. Be explicit in your desire to learn. Many people are pleased to share their expertise and experience.

What to Write About

Beginning writers sometimes feel they have nothing to say. But, virtually everyone has felt on reading someone else's work, "I could say that better," or has been told, "That was really a good presentation, you ought to publish it," or has been asked, "May I have a copy of the paper you gave at the ... meetings?" (which it turns out you only partially wrote or wrote but did not think enough of to revise and submit for publication). As a family medicine educator in a complex field, there are a variety of writing opportunities. Write about what to do, where to do it, how to do it, who should do it, when to do it, what new or old knowledge is needed to do it, or what happened in an unusual case (the case study).

Finding Time to Write

Although academic work often requires working longer than a 40-hour week, it is unrealistic to assume or for others to expect that all writing will be done on one's own time. If publishing is an expected part of the job, then time should be allowed for it. It may be more difficult to renegotiate for such time on one's current job than to negotiate for it on a new one, but it is possible. Some departments have the policy that 10–20% of faculty time is for "personal growth and development." That may not sound like much, but it is a half or a full day a week. If time is available or can be made available periodically, but is often, magically, taken up with other activities, another approach may be necessary. You may need to be firm with yourself (after all, how can you consistently find time to answer correspondence but not to write an article?), reorganize your schedule, and inform the secretarial staff not to make appointments for you during the time you have set aside. You may then need to close your office door leaving instructions not to be disturbed, write at home and then come into the office, or go to the library or a lab to work away from other demands on your time. Even some professional writers have a special office which they use for writing. Therefore, it is not strange for you to seek out some special place in which to write.

Other writers do use some of their own time for writing. They rise early and write for an hour before they start on the rest of their daily activities. It is in this way that surgeon William Nolan started his writing career. William Buckley does work on his detective stories as distinct from his newspaper column and editorial duties in time he has set aside in this way. Still others find that they work best when they can periodically work almost nonstop on a weekend or late into the night until they have a first draft. The point is that one does not need a large block of time but some time on a fairly consistent basis that is free from distractions and interruptions. In this way it is possible to start the writing process and keep it going. In finding this time you may need to decide what is the most productive time of the day for you to do creative work versus other activities.

How and How Much to "Write"

Although the focus has been *writing* a draft, alternatively, a draft can be dictated or discussed with a colleague, tape-recorded, and then transcribed. The point is somehow to get something on paper which you can then revise.

There are a number of methods of getting things on paper. These include using legal or regular size pads of paper and writing in longhand on every second or third line so that additional thoughts or corrections can be added. Those who type may triple space their work. It is generally better just to write on one side of the paper so if you later want to cut the work up and paste it together in another way, it is easier to do this. Once your thoughts are somehow translated to paper, it is easier to begin to see what else needs to be added, or how things can be better organized.

Another fallacy about writing is how much progress is made in one sitting. This may vary from day to day, but many professional writers consider a good day's work to be 5 to 10 pages of, often, triple-spaced text. This is not, generally speaking, final copy but a draft that will then need to be revised. You may feel that you are not making any progress because it seems to take so long to write a few pages. You may, however, be expecting more from yourself than humanly possible at any one writing stint. Although 5 to 10 pages may not seem like much for 1 day, in 5 writing sessions, that is 25 to 50 pages. Since many journal articles, when submitted, are only 10 to 20 double-spaced typewritten pages, those 25 to 50 pages could be 1 to 5 drafts of what you need.

Delaying Tactics

When faced with actually starting to write, writers often find other tasks begin to gain appeal. These may range from answering letters, cleaning the desk, making a few telephone calls, or even paying bills. Authors often talk of delaying tactics or rituals, such as sharpening a handful of pencils, that they go through before starting to write. Some of these rituals make the environment more comfortable for beginning to write. Unless they prevent you from starting to write, it is perhaps better to be tolerant of these foibles and recognize that others, too, do them.

Part of the problem in beginning is that we expect too much of ourselves, not only in terms of the amount of writing produced but also in its initial quality. It helps to keep in mind that writing *is a process* that involves successive efforts or approximations of what you want to say. For example, Tichy (1966) in a handbook on technical writing goes so far as to discuss what to focus upon in the *fourth* and *fifth* or successive revisions. (By these drafts, he suggests you should be focusing on deleting unnecessary words and sentences, and developing a better writing style.) If you can keep in mind that you do not have to and, in fact, are unlikely to "get it right" the first time you write it, this, too, can make starting easier.

Outlining: Its Pros and Cons

Well, if you have a topic, have delayed as long as possible, but finally feel no choice but to start, never fear, it is possible to get bogged down here. Where and how should you start? There are several approaches to this. These are "the-outline-what-you-are-going-to-do" and "the-forget-the-outline-just-start" schools of thought.

More people have been scared away from writing by Mrs. Grinch, their (grade school/high school/college) teacher and her rigid rules for Roman numeral outlines. Under these circumstances you may prefer to ignore outlining. Alternatively, you can think of outlining more open-mindedly than Mrs. Grinch did: It is a method of providing some skeleton or structure for organizing your thoughts. Since nobody but you will see your outline, it does not matter if you do not have at least two subjects under each heading or other dreaded failures in outlining. An "outline" can also be 3 × 5 cards or sheets of paper which you can try putting together in different kinds of order to see how your thoughts fit together. It can be phrases, lists of things you want to include, an abstract, sentences, paragraphs, or a tape-recorded discussion with a colleague. An outline is a method of describing what you want to do. It also serves as a jog to your memory if you have to stop writing or are interrupted. You then have a method of remembering where you were and ensuring that you did not, in the interim, forget something you wanted to include.

The forget-the-outline-school of thought suggests that you just start writing, even if you have to throw out the first paragraph or page of your work. Like a pump, writing often needs to be primed. Using this approach, you are urged to write as much as you can think of even if it initially seems unrelated to your topic. Do not worry about format, references, or pieces of information you have forgotten. Just write. Your jottings do not have to be complete sentences, logically related, or in the "correct" order. After you have a first draft, you can then go back and begin to fill in the blanks.

Another recommendation: Even when you have an outline, start where you want. This may be the part that is most interesting to you, easiest to write, or even the conclusion. The most important point is IT DOES NOT HAVE TO BE THE BEGINNING. Writing a beginning can be hard.

Sometimes this is because you may not know what the beginning is until you have a clearer notion of what you are trying to say. If beginnings are a real bugaboo, Tichy[1] reports that some people keep a handy reference list of different kinds of beginnings which they refer to in order to start. While this helps those who must begin at the beginning, it also leads to more variety and a more eye-catching repertoire of writing styles.

If you are starting work on a long composition, former *JAMA* editor Lester King (1978) suggests that rather than waiting until you have completed all your preparations and research, start writing 200- to 500-word preliminary segments as ideas come to mind. By writing in segments you not only begin to put some order to your thoughts, but also make starting less of a major problem.

Getting Stuck

Sometimes an author has been reading and thinking about a topic for long enough that, once started, he or she has little difficulty in writing. More commonly writing comes in fits and starts. Ideas will flow smoothly and then become bogged down. Some of the difficulties writers encounter are related to the dynamics of the creative process and others to personal psychological issues. In this section we shall examine both of these topics.

Some Technical Suggestions

It is somewhat heartening to know that getting stuck is a common enough problem, that techniques have developed to move around, through, or over writing blocks. Among these techniques are the following:

> Try brainstorming. Do not worry about turning out polished sentences, just write down as many ideas as possible. Follow brainstorming rules: Do not be critical of your ideas; be as freewheeling in your thoughts as you can be; think up as many things as possible, and, wherever possible, try to combine and improve upon your ideas (Stein, 1974:210).

---

[1]Tichy (1966) gives examples of the following types of beginnings: a summary of the content to follow, the scope of the paper, the point of view to be taken, specific details to catch the reader's attention, the purpose of the work, the plan of development to be followed, statement of the problem, review of background to the problem, a quotation, a question, statement of how interesting the topic is, comparison and contrast, defining and classifying the topic, an illustration or example of the subject to follow, setting up an argument to be demolished, an action focus, a forecast and hypothesis, wit or humor, or any combination of the above.

Use WIRMI in order to develop a more concise statement of your point. Switch from writing in standard English to talking to yourself: "What *I Really Mean Is.* . . . " (Flower, 1981).

"Satisfice." This coined term means "to accept an adequate, but imperfect, expression or idea in order to get on with more important problems (Flower, 1981:39). Do not worry about the structure of what you are writing. Instead, use phrases like "And another thing" or "The thing of it is . . . " just to keep your writing moving forward (Elbow, 1973).

Draw diagrams of what you are trying to say or make lists of phrases. Try using metaphors, analogies, examples of what you mean, or comparisons and contrasts of key ideas (Elbow, 1973; Flower, 1981).

Go over your notes again and jot down what they bring to mind. You may discover you have forgotten to include a key point or be able to see some connection that escaped you earlier.

Consider whether you are trying to cover too much in just one paper. The paper may represent competing thoughts and directions that would be better stated by being split in two.

Reread what you have written to see if that gives you some clues of what to do next. Beware, however, of becoming bogged down in rewriting. The aim is to immerse yourself in your argument, not to worry about its structure.

Keep the pen moving. Even if you normally type, King (1978) suggests switching to a pencil and copying over a relevant note, a thought from an earlier draft, or the last couple of sentences written before you became blocked. As you do this, change a word or phrase, no matter how minor. On your next attempt, try a bigger variation. These changes will eventually produce a new thought.

Try another variation of this approach. Kerrigan (1979) recommends a process by which you expand upon jotted phrases or sentences to flesh out your writing. Write a sentence outline, then write two sentences about each of these sentences. Next, write a paragraph about each of the sentences in step two. After this he suggests adding more concrete details and transitions.

Let the problem "cook" or simmer for a while in your mind. It may be that the process of synthesis is not complete yet. In fact, psychiatrist Lawrence Kubie (1967) reported that he did some of his "cooking" on "automatic pilot." He found it useful to write late into the evening until he reached a point where he became stuck. He then went to sleep and found that his unconscious often worked on the problem.

He might awaken in the middle of the night or in the morning with the solution. He cautions that if an idea comes to you in this way, write it down. Otherwise it is likely to flit away.

Ask a colleague for help. Explain what you are trying to do and where you are having trouble. The two of you may be able to see the fallacy or a way around the block. Brainstorm with this person to think of other approaches. Take notes, work on a blackboard, or tape-record the conversation so that you do not lose the important points.

Use a 10-minute "free-writing" exercise (Elbow, 1973). Write whatever is in your head, no matter how nonsensical or illogical. Since *something* is keeping you from writing, see if you can let it out so you can get back to your topic.

Collect examples of approaches for handling various thorny structural problems such as how to set up a complex statistical table. Then, if how to say or display something becomes a seemingly overwhelming block, you have a file of examples of what other people have done to solve similar problems.

Write, "I can't think of it now" or "Fix later" and go on to what is easier to do. This may work if you are not totally blocked but find yourself struggling over a particular section.

Switch to working on another chapter or article, or turn to another task altogether and start again the next day. Sometimes nothing helps but a little distance from the problem.

Pretend you have a public presentation to make. You have half an hour. Although your talk is not prepared as you would like, you have to talk anyway. Time yourself as you force yourself to write down what the project is about. As you go along, the focus may become clearer (Elbow, 1973).

Outline what you are trying to say. Even if you did an earlier outline, re-do it now to see what you have actually said. King (1978) advocates summarizing each paragraph into a sentence. This cuts out the superflous material and helps to refocus your writing.

What all these suggestions have in common is attacking the writing block from different angles, not letting ourselves become bogged down, overwhelmed, or stymied. Getting stuck happens. It is part of the creative process, a way in which the mind works over a problem, processing information, and recombining it.

Self-Awareness

What if, after trying these suggestions, you still get stuck and get stuck badly? At this point a little introspection may be in order. For example, do you dislike dictums of any kind and see "publish or perish" as another "should" or "ought" at which you balk? It is hard to sort out these issues, but if underneath it all you really do find writing at least occassionally enjoyable or interesting or if you are pleased or think you would be pleased when your work is finally published, you can bring your own reasons for writing to the fore and downplay the external pressures.

Those who write about creativity or writing note that a writer needs self-esteem, confidence, or self-assurance. The converse, feeling inferior, can produce a block. We may feel our work is inferior to that of others, that we cannot say what we want as well as others, or that it will surely be found wanting. It may feel too risky to lay one's *self* open to criticism. Although writing comes from you, it is not the same as you. It helps to remember that criticism of your work is not the same as criticism of your self.

A writer can become stuck because of not wanting to be or appear to be too aggressive or competitive as a result of stating his or her case strongly. On the other hand, writing may be a way of being assertive for those who are not generally so. It may be a way of venting strong emotions that would not be expressed otherwise. An author may vacillate between these two positions. Unless a writer becomes aware of this possibility, he or she may constantly fight letting these emotions see the light of day in whatever their transmuted form. Such concerns can very effectively keep a person from writing.

Writers may become enamoured of their words and balk at deleting material or become too focused on making a point, even when the data are pointing in another direction. More importantly, a writer may be too attached to the topic to be able to separate him- or herself enough from it in order to work on it. Since the topics we write about, even in a scientific setting, are often some transmutation of our own experiences and concerns, unless some of the personal basis of these writing choices are clear, an author may become stuck.

Still other blocks may be related to personality type (Storr, 1972). An obsessive/compulsive may use writing as a way to be free of outside controls or to fit together disparate facts into a neater whole, but at the same time may struggle to maintain so much control that he or she becomes stuck. As we have seen, not allowing oneself enough spontaneity is antithetical to being able to write freely. Others may use writing to avoid becoming close to people or as a way to retain some degree of detachment from them.

Getting Finished

Why is it that sometimes you have completed several drafts of a paper but have still not submitted it for publication? One major possibility is perfectionism, a compulsive need to find one more reference, do one more statistical test, or rewrite some section of the paper just once more. Often this quest for perfection is due to fear of the consequences if the paper is found wanting.

As Alamshah (1972) suggests, it is also possible to have trouble completing an article because the fantasy of praise is more pleasing to contemplate than the threatening possibility of actually finishing the work and allowing others to examine it. There may also be a certain sense of control or power when only a small group of people know of your work informally. The world is then deprived of your superior work.

Self-conceit and lack of self-discipline can also produce the inability to finish a paper (Alamshah, 1972). For those for whom many tasks come easily, a certain kind of complacency may set in, a feeling that the need to write and rewrite does not apply to them. The result may be unclear writing, which enhances the likelihood that an article will be rejected for publication. The author in turn becomes discouraged and reluctant to try again. Be advised: First, that many authors' first articles are rejected, and, second, that the majority of articles eventually accepted for publication were initially sent back for often quite substantial revisions. Learn from the suggestions made by reviewers and the journal editor and try again.

One way to shorten the editorial review process is to ask a colleague to review your manuscript before you submit it. You need to find people who are able to review kindly and considerately but thoroughly. It does not help to have something reviewed by an uncritical reader, but, on the other hand, you do not want to be overly discouraged by a savage review [see DeBakey (1976) and chapter 10 of this book for some useful guidelines for reviewing papers]. In addition to local colleagues, consider asking others with similar research interests whom you have met at scientific meetings. You need to find supportive, informed critics.

Another method people use to finish their work is to set up personal deadlines and rewards even for subgoals: "I'll play tennis if I get this part done" or "I want to finish this before vacation." Elbow (1973) suggests if freezing-up is such a problem that one commonly is unable to finish on time, it may help to write a rough draft far in advance of the deadline. Even if it is not very good, it can then be revised to turn in by the deadline. This will also mean you have started your paper early enough to gather additional data if need be and to give your ideas a chance to "cook" a while.

Hiring an Editor

If you have a draft of your ideas and cannot seem to complete the paper, are having trouble cutting out material a publisher wants you to delete, or need help with grammar and punctuation, consider hiring an editor. He or she can rewrite your work for you. Some authors almost exclusively use this approach, once they have a draft of their ideas. Such services can even be used to search out references. Editorial assistance for technical writing is often available through the university library or the English department. Hiring an editor not only helps prepare your article but also allows you to learn from the changes the editor makes in your work so that you can write better in the future.

Writing Support Groups

Another spur to writing is what Elbow (1973) calls the teacherless writing class. A group of people interested in improving their ability to write meet weekly to try "free-writing" exercises and review one another's work. Another approach is that of an interdisciplinary group of medical faculty at the Texas Medical Branch at Galveston. They established a publication club to encourage writing (Meier, 1982). To participate, members must have presented or published at least one paper but have a total of 12 or fewer publications. The group meets every 6 weeks. The members provide encouragement and support for authors who have submitted articles and discuss research ideas, works in progress, completed projects ready to submit, and requirements for journal articles. In 2 years, the number of articles and book chapters published by group members increased 55%.

Word processors are a technical aid to finishing a piece of work. Materials can easily be added, deleted, or rearranged. This is a boon to the fussy writer and avoids long waits for retyping drafts. Commonly used references can also be typed in the reference format you use, stored in the word processor, and pulled from the master list as needed.

If All Else Fails . . .

If acceptance of the processual nature of writing, techniques, introspection, rewards, or advice from others do not help you to complete your writing, several other possibilities need to be examined. It may be that you really, absolutely, do not want to write, do not like your work, and fundamentally are not committed to it. As Alamshah (1972:112) notes, "the hope of being creative demands what we commonly call commitment. . . . Hence, absence of commitment functions as a blockage to creativity." It is hard to write without a commitment to the task.

You may decide you would rather have a position in which you can spend more time on other tasks, such as teaching or patient care. Although career changes or changes in career direction are difficult, they are not impossible.

If you want to write but find that you cannot or that it is much more anxiety provoking and difficult than you feel it should be, professional help may be needed (Stein, 1974). Such help might also be called for if there are such serious problems in other areas of one'e life that they make it hard to concentrate or if one could write at one point but no longer can.

Conclusion

This review of methods of handling writing problems suggests a two-pronged attack. First, it helps to recognize that creativity, and writing as a specific form of it, is a *process*. Once appropriate preparations have been made through reading or gathering empirical data and, possibly, outlining, a writer still may not know how the material will actually coalesce until he or she begins to write. It helps to remember that the process of combination and recombination of material takes time. This means writing sessions when words come smoothly and others when it feels like you are mired in mud and sinking fast. It means multiple drafts, false leads, additions, deletions, and corrections. Once we accept that these are normal, natural parts of the writing process, our impatience with what may seem like snail-like progress can be reduced. At the same time, a variety of techniques have been developed to help the writing process along and to avoid becoming stymied. They work.

The second prong of the attack on writing blocks is a more personal one. It involves developing greater self-awareness of what are some of the points at which we become stuck. These are much more individual. But, until we have given some serious thought as to *why* it is so hard to start, *why* we sometimes become stuck so badly, or *why* it is so hard to finish a paper, these unknown, or only dimly known forces, not us, may control our writing. They do not have to do so.

Faculty Development Activities

(1) You need to choose your best time for your writing. When are you most creative—in the mornings, evenings, etc.? Combine your writing activities with your unique creative times—no one else can tell you when is your best time to write.

(2) Once you have decided when your most productive times are, keep a time log for 1 week. This will show you how you are currently spending your time. Outline a plan to place time(s) for writing in your weekly schedule. It may be helpful to divide your writing activities into categories—administrative, educational, research articles, etc.

(3) Organize a procedure to assure undisturbed, scheduled time for writing. A couple of suggestions:
  (a) Place a "do not disturb" sign on your door and have your secretary hold all calls.
  (b) Find a special place to write: at home, the library, or hospital.

(4) Procrastination is a delaying tactic many people use. What rituals do you use to avoid writing? If they seriously hinder your production, outline a plan to eliminate these rituals.

(5) List the pros and cons of writing from an outline. As you write your list you will become clearer as to your own personal preferences.

(6) Review the technical suggestions in this chapter regarding "Getting Stuck." If these do not help, try some introspection by asking yourself "Why am I afraid to write?"

Acknowledgments

I am grateful to Jason Chao, George Drake, James Kitson, Robert Like, Justin Phillips, Joseph Raj, and L. Edwin Speagle for their helpful comments on earlier versions of this paper.

References

Alamshah WH. Blockages to creativity. J Creative Behavior 1972;6:105–13.

Berkov W, Baker R. Coming of age in hard times. The Plain Dealer 1982 Oct 25:D2(col 1).

DeBakey L. The scientific journal: editorial policies and practices. St. Louis: CV Mosby, 1976.

Elbow P. Writing without teachers. New York: Oxford University Press, 1973.

Flower L. Problem-solving strategies for writing. New York: Harcourt, Brace, Jovanovich, 1981.

Kerrigan WJ. Writing to the point: six basic steps. 2nd ed. New York: Harcourt, Brace, Jovanovich, 1979.

King LS. Why not say it clearly: A guide to scientific writing. Boston: Little, Brown and Co., 1978.

Kubie LS. Blocks to creativity. In: Mooney RL, Razik T, eds. Explorations in creativity. New York: Harper and Row, 1967:33–42.

Luthe W. Creativity mobilization technique. New York: Grune and Stratton, 1976.

Maslow AA. The creative attitude. In: Mooney RL, Razik T, eds. Explorations in creativity. New York: Harper and Row, 1967:43–54.

Meier RS. Encouraging writing in family medicine. Fam Med XIV 1982;4:26ff.

Plimpton G. ed. Writers at work: the Paris review interviews, second series. New York: Viking Press, 1963. Cited in: Tichy HJ. Effective writing for engineers, managers, scientists. New York: John Wiley, 1966.

Stein MI. Stimulating creativity Vol. I: Individual procedures. New York: Academic Press, 1974.

Storr A. The dynamics of creation. New York: Atheneum, 1972.

Tichy HJ. Effective writing for engineers, managers, scientists. New York: John Wiley, 1966.

Wallas, G. The art of thought. New York: Harcourt, Brace, 1926. Cited in: Flower L. Problem-solving strategies for writing. New York: Harcourt, Brace, Jovanovich, 1981.

Part II

Writing for Publication

Chapter 3

Writing a Medical Article

Joseph E. Scherger and Robert B. Taylor

Medical writing for publication is done for various purposes: The publication of original work is integral to an academic career, allows an individual to contribute to the growing body of medical literature, and serves as a vehicle for the worldwide communication of medical information. Medical writing is also a skill, one which, like performing an obstetrical delivery or counseling a dysfunctional family, requires training and practice to be mastered.

Medical writing may be considered one of the final steps in conducting a research study and should be undertaken with the same diligence as other steps of the project. The results of outstanding research or the description of an excellent educational program may fail to be published if written poorly.

For the experienced medical writer, following a methodical, stepwise approach to writing a medical article will increase the chances of successful publication. The following will describe 10 steps in writing a medical article. The steps are presented as a workbook which may assist in the writing of an article and as a review for assessment of subsequent writing efforts. A period of time is suggested for each step to illustrate the relative effort that may be required.

More than one author may be involved with the writing of an article. While any of the following steps may be a shared activity, generally one author takes responsibility for writing the first draft and the other(s) for additions and revision. The authors should agree ahead of time as to their respective responsibilities and who will be the primary author of the article.

Conceptualize the Subject of the Article (1–3 Days)

Careful planning before beginning to write greatly enhances the flow of words. Ask: "What am I trying to say in this article?" When the answer to this question is clear in your mind, write a topic sentence or working title. Limit the subject and be as specific as possible in order to bring into focus what will be reported in the article. The following are examples of broad topic areas which should be limited before writing:

Broad: Quality of care in a community hospital.
Specific: Peer review using retrospective audits in a community hospital.
More Specific: Peer review using a retrospective audit of coronary care in a community hospital.

Broad: What is wrong with tenure in medical education?
Specific: The impact of tenure on productivity among medical school faculty.
More Specific: The impact of tenure on research activity among faculty in a clinical department.

Review the Literature (1–2 Weeks)

Defining the topic of the article simplifies the next step, which is to review the medical literature. A medical librarian, acting as an expert consultant to the writer, can be very helpful in acquiring the appropriate background material.

A computerized search of the recent literature is generally the best way to begin. Index Medicus, FAMLI (specific articles for *Family Medicine*), or the Index and Table of Contents of selected journals may also be used to find current articles on the chosen subject. The bibliography of these articles may be useful in identifying the earlier background literature.

After the published literature on the subject has been identified and read, a good idea may be to telephone a known expert to discuss current thinking and inquire regarding unpublished information.

After reading the medical literature, the goals and subject of the article should be reconsidered. A change in the research hypothesis or in the article concept may be appropriate, and it is much easier to do so at this stage than after several rejections of a finished manuscript.

The final step in the literature review is to select potential references and categorize them according to points to be covered in the article.

Select the Appropriate Readership and Journal (1 Day)

Selecting an audience for the article helps to focus the writing effort. Look through recent issues of selected journals giving attention to topics, style, format, and length of articles. Make a provisional decision as to your target journal with a list of alternative publications if the manuscript is rejected. Journals which are commonly considered by family medicine authors include:

Family Medicine (published by STFM)

The Journal of Family Practice

American Family Physician

The Journal of Family Practice Research

The Journal of the American Medical Association (*JAMA*)

The Journal of Medical Education

Medical Care

Medical Education

Local, state, or regional publications

Study the Instructions to Authors for the journal selected for submission. Most publications (including *Family Medicine*) subscribe to the "Uniform Requirements for Manuscripts Submitted to Biomedical Journals" (see Appendix IV).

Organize and Outline the Content of the Article (1 Week)

The writing process should begin with an outline. Organize notes, tables, figures, and references under headings suitable for the topic. Discard material that does not fit rather than attempting to find a spot to "get it in."

For a research article the usual headings are:

Introduction

Methods

Results (including tables and figures)

Discussion

Abstract/Summary

References

For most other types of medical articles, the general outline may be:

Introduction/Background

Body

Discussion

Summary/Abstract

References

The outline for an article may be suggested by the concept, for example:

New Drugs Used to Treat Congestive Heart Failure

Pneumocystis carinii Pneumonia: Report of Three Cases and Discussion

How to Select a Computer for Your Office

The outline is a final opportunity to clarify the topic and content of the article. As you develop the outline, you will find that most headings logically break down into subheadings. Within each of these subheadings, think of general statements supported by data from your research or the literature.

Select a Title (1 Day)

A provisional title is a good place to start writing since it is a further refinement of the topic sentence. The title sets the tone for the content to follow.

The title should state what the article is about. It should be precise, original, and scholarly, incorporating key words that will clearly identify your article for the reader. The medical author should avoid catchy phrases and variations of popular titles. Shorten or divide the title rather than have a long sentence. The title should not indicate a specific locale unless necessary.

Examples of poor titles with improvements are:

To Treat or Not to Treat: The Dilemma of Trichomoniasis in Pregnancy. (Too long, mimics a well-known phrase.)

Better: Trichomonas Infection in Pregnancy: A Theraputic Dilemma

The Utilization of a Nurse Practitioner in the University of Washington Family Practice Residency with a Description of the Role and a Study of the Impact on the Continuity of the Relationship between the Patient and Practitioner.
(Too long, needs to be divided, local reference detracts.)

Better: A Nurse Practitioner in a Family Practice Residency: Role Description and Impact on the Practitioner-Patient Relationship.

Write the First Draft (1–2 Weeks)

Begin writing the text without hesitation. Start with the section of the article that seems the easiest. For a research article, the Methods and the Results sections (with preparation of the tables and figures) are often done first.

Do not confuse writing, a creative activity, with revising, an editorial function. The first draft should be written as smoothly and rapidly as possible, with more attention to the content and flow of ideas than to the details of writing style.

The contents of each section of a research article follows.

Introduction

The first sentence should arouse the reader's interest in the report that follows. Avoid truisms such as: "Family medicine is a new and exciting discipline," or "The sedative effect of antihistamines is well known."

The first sentence should precisely describe the subject of the article, or the issues from which the subject derives, and the first paragraph should expand upon this sentence.

The flow of paragraphs in the Introduction may be as follows:

(1) The subject, the issues of the article (or study);
(2) A description of how previous works related to the subject;
(3) The purpose and setting for the article (or study), the "research questions" to be answered.

Avoid using too global a background, such as reviewing the history of family medicine. Avoid an early reference to the local setting, which may limit the scope and breadth of interest in the article.

Methods

Clearly state how the study was done in sufficient detail so that it could be replicated. The reader should be told:

(1) The where and when of the study;
(2) How the subjects in the study were selected and if there were any exclusions;
(3) What information was sought and how it was collected;
(4) Any factors which might have limited or biased the selection of subjects or collection of data;

(5) What statistical methods were used and, if other than standard procedures, why they were selected.

Results

This section contains the pertinent data, not necessarily all of the data obtained in the study, and it is often useful to review the research question as a guide to data selection. The results should be stated as facts without interpretive or qualifying information.

Although tables and figures are often the best way to present research data, they should be used judiciously because they occupy considerable space and are expensive to publish. Tables are chosen for data presentation; figures are used for data illustration. Each table or figure, with its legend, must be self-sufficient—that is, not dependent on the narrative for interpretation. They should supplement, not duplicate, the written text. Guidance with the preparation of tables and figures may be obtained from a statistician or medical artist, or from books in the Reference List.

Discussion

The flow of paragraphs in this section may be as follows:

(1) An interpretation of the results. The first sentence is important and should stimulate the reader to continue reading. Discuss the limitations or possible biases in the study. Be direct and avoid qualifying phrases such as: "it appears that..." or "our data suggest the possibility of..."
(2) A discussion of how the results relate to previously published articles; these are likely to have been mentioned in the Introduction.
(3) Generalizations or conclusions from the study and, if appropriate, suggestions for future research.

Abstract/Summary

An abstract is a factual summary of the article. For a research article, it should contain a statement of the *purpose* of the study, the *results*, and the *conclusions* drawn. It is generally written in the past tense, and is often in the first person, e.g., "We examined the relationship of..."

Do not use phrases such as "the findings are described," or "the relationship is discussed," which require reading the article to obtain the information. Do not include background data such as the reasons for the study or references to the literature.

Most abstracts for medical journals contain four to five sentences and about 150 words.

References

For any references used, the original article should have been obtained and read during the review of the literature. References cited should be integral to the article, and not added as terminal appendages to the manuscript.

While writing the first draft, do not number the references since they are likely to change with revisions. Noting the first author and date in parentheses is adequate until the final draft.

For listing the references, use the style required by the journal. Be accurate and complete in recording authors' names, article or book title, volume number, pages, and date.

Write the First Revision (1 Week)

It has been said that good papers are not written, but rather rewritten. The primary author of the first draft should do the first revision. Review the manuscript for clarity, style, and accuracy. There should be a logical flow of ideas, without repetition, and material that is not pertinent to the main subject should be eliminated. Be sure that generalizations are supported by facts, and that the objectives of the paper are clearly stated and ultimately achieved.

At this stage, avoid any temptation to submit the manuscript for publication, since a rejection is almost certain.

Submit the Manuscript for Review by Selected Colleagues (1–2 Weeks)

Ask several colleagues to review the manuscript. Any co-authors who participated with the study should be involved, but do not limit the review to this group. Request that the reviewers be as objective and specific as possible. The best reviewer is someone with expertise in editing journal articles, who will provide honest criticism of the article's defects.

While the manuscript is with reviewers, the primary author should take a break from the project.

Write a Final Draft (1–3 Weeks)

After evaluating the comments of the reviewers, prepare another draft. Do not feel obligated to agree with or incorporate all of the reviewers' suggestions. The next revision may be returned for further comments to one or more of the reviewers, and certainly to all co-authors. Once you are satisfied that an excellent article has been written, a final draft is prepared according to the guidelines of the selected journal.

Submit the Paper for Publication (1 Day)

A brief transmittal letter to the editor of the journal should accompany the manuscript, with clear instructions telling whom the editor might write or call if questions arise. Although a brief statement about the article may be appropriate, avoid explaining or promoting the manuscript. The submission letter with the requested number of manuscript copies should be sent by first class mail in a strong manila envelope or a reinforced mailing bag. The author should keep a copy of the manuscript. If a letter of acknowledgment from the journal is not received within two weeks, you should contact the editorial office.

Submitting a carefully prepared manuscript for publication is a praiseworthy accomplishment. Receiving the comments from the journal reviewers about 6 weeks later may be a humbling experience—or a cause for celebration. If the above steps are followed, and if you are willing to further revise the manuscript according to the comments of the journal editors, the experience of writing for publication will often be successful.

Faculty Development Activities

(1) It is important to know your motivation(s) for writing. Some are clearly internal (i.e., you like to share your ideas with others) while others are external (i.e., you are expected to publish to get tenure). List your motivations both internal and external. Use these motivations to keep you writing.

(2) Read the letters to the editor in your favorite journals. Do they mainly contain medical information/conjecture or any other topic/opinion? Have you ever read an article and wanted to contribute additional information or a differing opinion? If so, next time that happens, sit down and write a brief, succinct reply using the principles in this chapter.

(3) After reading this chapter, outline the components (i.e, literature search, timeline, optimal resources) involved in the production of a case study, review of the literature, book chapter and a book. This outline will give you a clearer picture about the steps involved in writing each format.

References

Day RA. How to write and publish a scientific paper. Philadelphia: ISI Press, 1979.

Geyman JP, Bass MJ. Communication of results of research. J Fam Prac 1978;1:113–20.

Howie JW, Whimster WF, Paton A, et al. Writing and speaking in medicine. Br Med J 1976;3:1113–25.

Huth EJ. How to write and publish papers in the medical sciences. Philadelphia: ISI Press, 1982.

International Committee of Medical Journal Editors. Uniform requirements for manuscripts submitted to biomedical journals. Ann Int Med 1982;96 (Part 1):766–77.

King LS. Why not say it clearly: a guide to medical writing. Boston: Little, Brown and Co., 1978.

The Task Force on Professional Communication Skills of the Society of Teachers of Family Medicine. Written Communication in Family Medicine. Kansas City, Mo., STFM, 1984.

Chapter 4

Seeking Publication

General Issues and Tips for Letters to the Editor, Case Reports, Literature Reviews, and Book Chapters or Books

Pamela LaVigne

Having your writing published is the end point of a long journey. This chapter is a guidebook to the trip, describing several different destinations and including some general notes about traveling. It opens with an overview of seeking publication: why family medicine faculty write, where they send their writing, and what different kinds of pieces are published in journals and books. Next it discusses three issues basic to all writing for publication, from making a commitment to the writing, through reading, to revising. The concluding segment of this chapter provides pointers for composing (in ascending order of complexity) a letter to the editor, case report, literature review, and book chapter or book.

Seeking Publication: Why? Where? What?

Why write?

If you are like other family medicine writers, your reasons for seeking publication range widely. In my teaching and editorial consultations with them, family medicine faculty have mentioned the following reasons why they write for publication:

Advance the field	Secure tenure
Call for action	Share ideas

Present research	Get credit for work
Philosophize	Pass on anecdotes
Update information	Describe an event or activity
Review literature	Report a case
Earn income	Solicit comments
Generate discussion	Justify an action taken
Serve a political purpose	

Clearly, many motives fuel the urge to write, and you will probably find yourself responding to more than one in the process of preparing even a single piece.

Once you have the idea to write something for publication, your next questions invariably will concern *where* to publish and *what* type of piece to submit. A quick overview of family medicine publications reveals encouraging answers to both questions.

Where to Send Your Writing?

Publishing opportunities devoted expressly to family medicine topics abound. Periodicals include association-sponsored journals (*American Family Physician*—American Academy of Family Physicians and *Family Medicine*—Society of Teachers of Family Medicine), independent publications (*Journal of Family Practice, Family Practice Research Journal*), plus two forthcoming new titles (*Family Medicine Reports* and *Family Systems Medicine*). Book publication too is strong in family medicine. From the first major book in family medicine (Conn, et al., 1973) to the most recent (Taylor, 1983) numerous related texts and specialized books are available, offered by top medical, scientific, and textbook publishers (Gehlbach, 1982; Bland, 1980; Fabb et al., 1976). Besides these established avenues of publication for family medicine authors, conference proceedings also advance the creation of family medicine literature (Lipkin, Jr., et al., 1982; Currie, 1983).

What Kind of Writing?

As for what family medicine faculty write, besides books, consider the following types of articles found in medical journals:

Abstracts	Opinions/editorials
Research articles	Literature reviews
Book reviews	Special political sections
Case reports/Case series	History

Letters to the editor	Biography
Teaching articles	Brief communications
Techniques, how-tos	

The novice author in our field should note: Research is not always the topic. This point is made not to minimize the importance of research, but rather to encourage beginners with the reminder that many different topics appear in medical writing, and many topics are suitable for formats of various lengths, from letters to books.

Thus, you will join distinguished and ever more numerous company when you write for publication in family medicine. You also will enter a process characterized by difficulty as well as delight. So, before I describe how to organize several different kinds of writing, I want to discuss briefly the writing process as experienced by the individual author.

Recommendations for Writers

What I have to say next is based on my extensive experience as editor, writing coach, and instructor to family medicine teachers writing for publication. Though my clinical exposure comprises literally hundreds of manuscripts in our field, here I want to address not manuscript requirements but writer requirements. I have seen family medicine authors, myself included, grapple with similar issues time and again when writing for publication. For the benefit of budding and experienced writers alike, I want to consolidate and pass on here some of the lessons to be learned from that struggle.

These lessons can be distilled into three main observations and three corresponding recommendations for anyone contemplating writing for publication:

(1) Writing does not come easy, so deliberately decide if it is worth it to you.
(2) Reading is writing's companion process, so use your experience as a reader to guide your writing.
(3) Writing is an interaction with yourself, so expect to be surprised by your writing and to rewrite substantially.

These observations roughly parallel the stages of any writing project, and each is discussed separately below.

Is Writing Worth It to You?

My first recommendation to family medicine faculty writing for publication is: Decide where publications fit into your professional life. Making that decision means reflecting on your own interests and others' expectations.

First, what faculty role—service, teaching, research, administration—is most engaging to you? Your answer is important since publication carries a different weight in each. If you answer "research," publication must be an essential component of research activity. By contrast, practitioners who regard service as their most important role may feel little interest in, and even less incentive for, writing for publication.

Next, consider the setting in which you function as a faculty member. Is it primarily community based (like most STFM members), university affiliated, or a mix of both? The demands, support, and rewards for writing vary greatly across these settings. Even in a university setting, you must gauge how powerful the expectation is that family medicine faculty write for publication. At a major university with a reputation for research, publication is the coin of the realm for a faculty member. At a smaller or less research-oriented school, the expected and actual publishing performance of faculty may be quite different.

The decision to make writing for publication a significant portion of your professional life should be deliberately considered. Knowing both what aspect of your job is most meaningful to you and what is expected of you in terms of publication, then you can decide whether the payoff for writing is great enough, what topics you find most worth writing about should you decide it is, and where to submit your work.

Once you have made the decision to write for publication, throughout the entire writing process remember that you write for someone else to read. How reading and writing are related and how to incorporate an awareness of that connection into your own writing are discussed next.

Reading and Writing: Companion Processes

Reading is writing's companion process. For this reason, your experience as a reader provides valuable guidance for your practice as a writer. I make this point for the benefit of novice and experienced authors both—to encourage the former who think they are unprepared for this new task, and to encourage as well the latter, as a reminder that there is always room for improvement. By reading, I refer both to others' work which you consult and your own work which you reread to improve.

Reading others' work influences you as a writer in at least five ways.

(1) Reading in your field helps you stay abreast of scholarly activity and pertinent announcements, knowledge that keeps you from discrediting yourself by omission when you write.

(2) Going back to sources you have already read refreshes your memory even about a familiar topic and shores up the specific content of your own writing.

(3) Reading stimulates your creativity. It does this by exposing you to questions that authors themselves propose for further work as well as by promoting your own critiques, questions, and suggestions.

(4) Apart from providing, reviving, and prompting further development of information on a certain subject, reading also exposes you to examples of how things can be expressed, well or poorly. Your reading may turn up models of effective prose that you will want to save for inspiration or imitation later.

(5) Last, reading can directly influence your writing when the reading content addresses writing itself—writing tips, descriptions by other authors of how they work, etc.

Your reactions during the process of reading are worth remembering also as you organize your writing for someone else to read. Having been one yourself, you know that a reader is looking for something, usually pressed for time, not always attuned to subtlety. A reader has immediate reactions both to writing content and to style, reactions no less striking than if you were hearing the author's actual voice. And last, you also know that when you have to work too hard to understand what you are reading, you will probably stop trying.

How might these experiences as a reader apply to your efforts as a writer? They are useful in many ways from start to finish, as you will see.

Surprisingly often, authors overlook directing their writing to a particular reader. It is not unusual for me to finish reading a manuscript and have no clue as to who the intended reader is. So when you first organize your writing, begin by deciding whom you most want to reach. Then make rough judgments about that intended reader's knowledge vis-à-vis your own, and decide what angle on your subject would be most appealing to this reader. Keep in mind the advice given young journalists: Do not underestimate readers' intelligence, or overestimate their information. Are there aspects of your topic for which the ideal reader might require some orientation? What questions would you anticipate this reader asking? Look for ways to order your writing so that it reflects your awareness that a real person is being addressed.

This discussion so far has concerned your preparations for writing—consciously choosing to do it, and remembering that reading, both its content and its process, affords useful direction as you organize what you have to tell a reader. My final recommendation concerns all that you do after your first draft is completed.

Writing as Interaction with Yourself

If reading captures your interest, writing focuses it. Reading prompts thought, but writing stimulates and nurtures thought, pulling you beyond what you knew when you first sat down to write. Influential as reading is to your writing, reading alone will not make you a better writer. For that, you must, simply, write.

When you do, you will find that writing is self-guided instruction. Think about this for a moment. Rather than thinking of writing as a way of expressing what you already know, think of it as a process that will teach you more. The Big Surprise about any writing you will do is not that it is demanding, and takes time, and is different from just talking about the topic, but that through it you teach yourself—about the topic, and about thinking. Figuring out what you want to say, deciding how to say it, finding out as you are writing that it does not come out the way you planned, finding out later as you reread it that there is more to say than what you wrote ... or less ... or something completely different—this process reveals that writing is an engrossing, synergistic interaction. When you write, you keep changing your relationship to the writing: at one stage you write to record your thoughts; at the next you read to know them more clearly.

This recycling loop is writing's heart. It is the truth of the maxim: All good writing is rewriting. This observation has important implications for your writing. The bad news is that your first several drafts of any piece will not be complete, no matter what your expertise on the topic, your experience teaching in that area, or even your earlier writing about it. Do not be seduced by the typewritten page. Just because your thoughts now look tidy does not mean they are sufficiently steeped, and it certainly does not mean they are logical. Expect and search out the missing points, the mixed-up details. Take for granted that you know more than you were able to put into writing.

The good news is that, because writing is an interaction with yourself, you can learn to direct the interaction and thus improve your writing and thinking. Let me give you some suggestions for revising your work, beginning with some ideas that relate once again to your remembering the reader.

Set aside your manuscript for a week or more. Then, before rereading it, try to say in a sentence or two your main points—significant findings, important implications, whatever key messages you want to emphasize. Now look at your manuscript. Right away, do you alert readers to your purpose in writing? Will they find sentences clearly expressing the core of what you have to say at pertinent places throughout the manuscript? Recall too the likely reader questions you imagined as a way of shaping a rough early outline. Are they answered anywhere in your manuscript? When revising, your first concern should be making sure that you have said all that you intended to say.

I am continually surprised by a discrepancy I encounter during editorial consultations. It is this: The points that stand out in the manuscript usually sound only faintly the themes and emphasis given them when the author speaks face to face with me about the topic. Why this difference? Hesitation to exceed the data, a desire to avoid contaminating scholarship with opinion—these may be the reasons. More likely though the answer is simpler. The prose is unfinished, the author has not adequately revised it. Now it is true that you simply cannot think of everything when you are trying to get your ideas down on paper for the first time. But once you have a completed draft, you can look at its beginning, middle, and end to be sure each clearly relates to your purpose in the piece, to your intended audience, and to the other sections.

So in addition to testing content, you also should test your writing for its organization—by section, paragraph, sentence, and word. First, check the overall outline of your manuscript by simply looking at it. Does the length of a section reflect the emphasis you wish to give it, compared to other segments of the manuscript and to your main theme? Do you filibuster on some tangential topic, but limit a main point to a short sentence or two? Do you rely on the same sentence types to start and end sections and paragraphs? These problems of imbalance and repetition you can spot by rereading and correct through rewriting.

Here is another test for sections and paragraphs in your draft. When you reread, are you caught off guard by thoughts heading in one direction when the text veers in another? Does a paragraph just seem to quit, leaving you hanging without a transition into the next? Such reactions may indicate an idea begun but not developed or an idea misplaced in that part of the piece. Do you find yourself wanting to add, "For instance . . . " or "In other words . . . "? The urge to translate like this signals that something more is needed—more clarity, a verbal illustration perhaps, maybe the explanation should replace what you wrote originally.

At the level of the sentence and word, notice during your rereading if you stumble over a string of words. Read not only with an eye to your writing's arrangement but also with an ear to its sound, speed, and pattern. In fact, reading the whole manuscript aloud is a sure way to detect any problems along these lines. Pay particular attention to key terms. Is the meaning of each clear from context, or should each term be defined explicitly? If you believe that the meaning is self-evident from your writing, deliberately verify that assertion. Check that your use of significant terms is correct and consistent throughout the manuscript. Rodnick and Ransom's letter (1983) on the distinctions between common terms in family medicine is an excellent reminder of the importance of word meanings. Words are notoriously slippery in first drafts. Suspect them all.

So far I have emphasized ways you can interact with your writing to fortify its content and organization. Recalling that you write for someone else to read brings up a final area deserving attention during revision; your writing's impact. How does the piece come across to readers? In a word, how would they sum up its tone—formal/informal? arousing/undistinguished? polysyllabic/plain? Because much scholarly writing continues a tradition of stuffiness, I urge authors not to think of their work as "writing something up." "Writing up" suggests that simple language should be replaced by more high-blown prose. Instead I prefer to encourage authors to write down what was done, telling the story in language that sounds as though one person were addressing another of equal capacity for understanding. I advise them to think of their writing as a public launching of their work in a forum where the chances for confusion are as high as the number of readers, each of whom represents a compelling reason to speak directly and simply.

Although you can work on your own to refine your early drafts, eventually you must test your efforts on a few preview readers. Orient them to their task by asking them to judge the writing's completeness, accuracy, clarity, and "arousability." It helps to have someone well versed in your content area as one previewer, along with someone else whom you trust to provide a candid and constructive critique. Naturally, I believe an author's editor serves admirably in this latter capacity and is a valuable ally when you write for publication.

Having concluded these "travel tips" to the writer embarking on the journey of writing for publication, let us move on now for a closer look at specific destinations: the letter to the editor, case report, literature review, and book chapter or book.

Letters to the Editor

All journal editors welcome comments on their publication; not all editors publish them. Nonetheless, letters to the editor merit your consideration as a publication option: first, because letters and short pieces stand a better chance of being published than longer articles, and second, because published letters to the editor generally are titled and indexed, thus making them as retrievable as articles in the journal.

Where are letters to the editor found? The two largest circulation medical journals in the United States, *JAMA* and the *New England Journal of Medicine*, print many readers' letters in each issue. In British journals, such as *Lancet, British Medical Journal,* and *Journal of the Royal College of General Practitioners*, the correspondence section has long been a forum of lively discussion. Among family medicine journals a similar tradition is developing in the STFM periodical, *Family Medicine*.

What you will find in a journal's correspondence section ranges widely, from the critical to the poetical. Letters often are short versions of research articles, case reports, and case series. Sometimes you can follow the progress of a research study in the letters section: call for proposals, announcement of funding awards, development of national network and study protocol, preliminary findings. Finally, some letters can best be classified only as humorous, and even then they may provoke as much comment as more serious work.

To sum up these various possibilities, letters to the editor can be categorized as either one of the types: those containing medical information or medical conjecture, and those on just about any other topic (Roland, 1975). Though both types are minor works in terms of their length, they should not be considered minor in terms of care in writing.

Care should particularly be taken with the first type of letter, one about medical topics. The form of these letters should follow that of the longer versions of same (as directed below for case reports and in the preceeding chapter for research articles). As a matter of fact, since the format is similar whatever the length of the piece, from the outset you might consider producing only a letter-length version of your report, instead of a longer article. (Space is always a consideration in a scholarly journal, so whenever your work involves less than nationwide activity, you should consider any section *but* the journal's leading contribution as a suitable place for publishing your report.) Certainly you need not be offended if the editor suggests converting to a shorter piece. "It is a fact that almost any manuscript can be shortened significantly without loss of its message: remarkably often, half as long is twice as nice" (Roland, 1975:627).

To prepare the second type of letter, one of opinion, Thorne (1970) advises a four-part approach. First, state your subject. Then note your purpose in writing and point of view on the subject. Develop your points next, limiting yourself to strictly pertinent information and avoiding self-serving comments. Last, sum up your conclusions, and stop!

Not all readers will share the letter writer's opinion, of course, so editors are especially wary that a published opinion letter avoid any suggestion of libel. On this matter, "when in doubt, leave it out" is a good rule to follow.

As for the writing quality of the opinion letter, strive for eloquence ("or its more common cousin, clarity...") and brevity (Roland, 1975:627). When the subject warrants, prefer the "rapier of sarcasm [rather] than the bludgeon of abuse" (Thorne, 1970:61); an angry monologue usually sounds petty and contrived once in print.

A cover letter for the letter to the editor may be necessary under two circumstances: (1) to give the editor additional background information, such as when your comments relate to articles appearing in another journal that does not publish a letters section, and (2) to request anonymity for yourself should the letter be published.

Writing a letter to the editor offers an opportunity for publication while posing its own writing difficulties. Since letters are not refereed, a published letter does not carry the same weight in one's vitae as an article that has been through the filter of review. On the other hand, its short length makes a letter to the editor more manageable as a first form of publication. Further, since statements of opinion are acceptable in the journal's correspondence columns, a letter to the editor makes an appropriate vehicle for expressing personal viewpoints and reactions on matters large and small. To write briefly and well, however, is not as easy as the short length of the letter would imply. Likewise, crafting a well-rendered critique requires a careful hand and conservative approach.

Case Reports

A case report is a brief report alerting practitioners to something of immediate clinical interest. When exactly does a case warrant being written? Advice on making that decision comes from several journal editors (Nahum, 1979; Huth, 1982). Write a case report, they say, when by doing so you will

Address a clinical problem of value to significant numbers of readers of the intended journal

Report a unique occurrence

Note a recent development in the field

Point out an unexpected association of diseases

Describe unexpected developments in a disease course

Even more stringent requirements have been published by the *Archives of Internal Medicine* (Soffer, 1982). Its editors say a case report warrants printing only when it

Establishes new principles

Modifies currently accepted concepts

As a would-be author of a case report, be cautious about trusting either your own or your colleagues' judgment of the uniqueness of a case and hence its intrinsic worthiness of publication. Both can easily be off the mark, as Rubin (1979) notes. After being advised to prepare a case report on a patient with an abdominal pregnancy, then finding that over 300 citations on the topic already exist, she conceded "Cases are apparently defined as 'rare' and are reported when an individual practitioner has not observed the complication previously—not when a situation is infrequently encountered by the medical profession as a whole" (Rubin, 1979:96). An extensive literature search should precede any report of a "first case." And even finding no references isn't conclusive, since you may not have searched far enough or the similar problem might have been earlier described in different terms.

Diseases that are rarely encountered anywhere certainly qualify for case reports, of course. In fact, it has been suggested that an international network may be needed to better capture the infrequent reports of these diseases (Soffer, 1982). Case reports of practitioner's experience in recognizing early signs of symptoms of these diseases make the format especially valuable for that purpose.

A written case report presenting a clinical problem should include four components (Nahum, 1979):

(1) Description of pertinent details about the patient—history, physical exam, and lab findings, including reasons for omitting lab tests if such was the case
(2) Differential diagnoses considered and reasons for selecting the diagnosis chosen
(3) Preferred and actual management, including possible complications and alternative treatment
(4) Discussion vis-à-vis the literature on the subject of the case reported, including, as in the discussion section of a research article, previous findings both supporting and refuting your diagnosis and treatment

The introduction to these many details should be well chosen, beginning with the title. The opening paragraphs should summarize succinctly how the case came to your attention, its clinical highlights, and what makes it noteworthy, specifying the literature search or other efforts to generate evidence (Huth, 1982).

Case reports then require as much care in preparation as major articles, both in terms of composition as well as consideration of an appropriate publication for submission.

Literature Review

A literature review is a process through which a reviewer identifies, collects, and synthesizes information. When you conduct a literature review, you are simultaneously teacher and student in what is essentially self-directed continuing education. Reviewing the literature, in its simplest terms, means investigating a topic by identifying and reading printed sources of information about it. Doing this requires a systematic approach and an unusually thorough exploration. Results of the review may be reported as part of a larger work such as a proposal or research article, or this process may result in a report that stands alone. This section focuses on the freestanding literature review.

A literature review serves varied purposes. Ladas (1980:597–598) notes four reasons for summarizing research:

(1) To reveal flaws in the previous work and recommend improvements
(2) To establish the academic rigor of both the research and the field
(3) To produce findings that will influence policy
(4) To reach conclusions for applied use

Cooper (1982:292), citing Jackson, also lists four purposes of a review of research:

(1) To size up new substantive or methodological developments in a field
(2) To verify or develop theory
(3) To synthesize knowledge from different lines of research
(4) To infer generalizations about substantive issues from a set of studies directly bearing on those issues

In addition to producing findings that benefit a discipline, you will enjoy immediate benefits from conducting a literature review as well (Moo-Dodge and Bland, 1981). Along with learning what is known about the subject, the reviewer learns what is not known. Earlier researchers may even have recommended areas for more study. Thus a literature review helps the researcher delineate a specific question for further work. Besides generating ideas for what to study, the literature review can also suggest how to study a question. Yet a third benefit to researchers is finding a preponderance of evidence to support a clinical decision.

Conducting a Literature Review

How should you conduct a proper literature review, one meeting the criteria of our opening definition: a systematic, unusually thorough investigation? Very conscientiously is the general answer. More specifically, you must learn to use the library and its resources: reference librarians, indexes, reference volumes, computerized data bases, and so forth. Though space does not permit even a short introduction to these here, several helpful articles exist and should be consulted before you begin conducting a review of the literature (Moo-Dodge and Bland, 1981; Stoan, 1982; Beatty, 1979).

Writing a Literature Review

Recall that the literature review being discussed here is a freestanding one, written expressly as its own end, hence considerably longer and more detailed than the selected references mentioned in a research article. Finding and synthesizing the references that comprise the review are forms of research called review research (Cooper, 1982). Thus, presenting the findings of such research might be done in the traditional format for research reports: the IMRAD structure. Discussed more fully in the previous chapter, IMRAD order refers to the conventional parts of a research article: Introduction, Materials and Methods, Results, and Discussion. What belongs where in a literature review organized according to this outline is explained next.

Introduction

Here you state the purpose of your review: finding an answer to a clinical problem, examining methods used to investigate a question, perhaps searching for the foundations or dimensions of theory. If your purpose lends itself to such distinctions, spell out both the conceptual and the operational definitions guiding your search in the Introduction.

Materials and Methods

Just as you would do when reporting descriptive or experimental work, in the Methods section you must spell out the steps you took to uncover literature for your review and exactly what sorts of literature you found: articles, books, theses, monographs, dissertations, etc. (some reviews also might include audiovisual materials). Thus in this section you should state what information sources you examined, such as print indexes and computerized data bases. For each, note what time period the source covered, the key words or other descriptors you used, and when in real time you were conducting these investigations. If possible, you should decide, before starting your search, any criteria for excluding literature found from literature read. Whether this decision is made in advance or in process, the exclusionary criteria should be stated in the Methods section.

Results

This section of a literature review is least amenable to prescription, since analysis is the core of a literature review, and the results of analysis, which should dictate the organization of this section, are entirely content dependent. Nonetheless, some general guidelines can be suggested. You might begin with a brief topical review that highlights pioneering or landmark work, summarizes major findings, and describes current work. Depending on your unique purpose, you may have to note variations in terms: the same terms defined in different ways, or different terms meaning essentially the same thing. You may need to introduce your own neutral terminology for the sake of comparison. You may describe methods typically used in your area of investigation, noting variations and critiquing them, if such is relevant to your purpose. You should describe the characteristics of the literature you examined. You must also describe sample characteristics of individuals in the studies reviewed, noting missing as well as overrepresented samples.

The rules of inference you applied to studies reviewed should be explicitly stated, and quantified if at all possible. Be careful to distinguish inferences made by authors of reviewed studies from those you make yourself on the basis of the overall review.

The person conducting review research wants to present information of value, depending on the review's purpose, either for its clinical significance or for its theoretical significance. Thus the reviewer struggles continually with the question of how much detail to report. Although this thoughtfulness is praiseworthy, basically you can never know for sure what is safe to leave out in reporting results of review research (Cooper, 1982:300).

Discussion

After the probably expansive display of your literature review results in the preceding section, here you are allowed to pronounce your inferred conclusions. This is the place to propose a theory, if such was your purpose, providing sufficient support for it was demonstrated in the Results section. Here too is the place to suggest areas for further study and perhaps methods to use as well.

The activities a literature review entails are critical to all scholarly work. A published literature review demonstrates the inseparable combination of reading and writing. It exemplifies the self-directed learning that is the heart of scholarship. And it is a generous contribution to a discipline, advancing its practitioners' understanding of their field. For all these reasons then, preparing a literature review for publication demands the highest standards of intellectual rigor and integrity from you.

Book Chapters and Books

Book chapters and entire books are an exciting development in any author's career, usually undertaken after the writer has had considerable experience in organizing and presenting material as well as writing for publication. In this final section I will describe various types of books, discuss two different roles authors play in preparing a book, and make specific suggestions for carrying out the responsibilities of each.

When you set out to write a book, your efforts could create a number of products: a collected work such as a yearbook, proceedings, text, or anthology; specialized book; or trade book. Let us define each.

Those in medicine, education, and many other professions look forward to the appearance of the latest *yearbook* in their field, which provides an annual update or review on topics of current interest. The yearbook's components are commissioned especially for the book and written primarily for members of a profession. Though often published by the professional association itself, yearbooks are also produced by publishing firms, as is the case with the *Yearbook of Family Medicine*.

A *proceedings* publishes some (rarely all) of the papers presented at a conference or meeting, again often sponsored by a professional organization. A special note: A proceedings runs the danger of being the most inconsistent of all collected works because conference presentations are solicited according to a broad general theme, not a specific book outline, hence proceedings selections may yield uneven coverage on a topic. Because of their appeal to special groups, yearbooks and proceedings are usually sold directly to them, rarely through bookstores.

Unlike both a yearbook and proceedings, an *anthology* consists of previously published work collected in one source. Though new material sometimes is written expressly for the anthology, it usually is limited to short introductory or biographical material about components and contributors. The anthology compiler is generally one person who approaches a publisher with specific selections in mind.

A textbook, which also collects information from various sources, highlights the history and research on a topic to introduce students to the topic. Though it may contain excerpts from others' works, a textbook generally paraphrases and condenses to cover the sweep of a topic, rather than its depth. The anthology and textbook would be available in a university or medical bookstore.

Besides the collected works just described, family medicine authors also might consider producing a specialized book or a trade book. A specialized book, also known as a technical publication, monograph, or scholarly work, is distinguished by the sophisticated level of its content. Since the specialized book is written for an author's colleagues and peers, it does not need to be as comprehensive as a text on the topic, nor as comprehensible as a book written for the general public. Titles in this latter category are called trade books—popular books on serious subjects. In medicine, education, and psychology, they are nonfiction works on provocative topics, written for the literate general reader. Trade books fall somewhere between specialized books and texts. A commercial publisher typically publishes specialized and trade books, and they are usually available in good general bookstores.

As an aspiring author of a book chapter, you could either be a contributor asked to supply a portion of the book or the book's initiator—compiler, editor, or author. This progression—from invitee to invitor—reflects increasing levels of responsibility which are outlined below.

When You Are a Book's Contributor

Being asked to contribute a section or more to a larger work is a sound first break into writing a book. But how does that invitation come about? William Van Til, in his book *Writing for Professional Publication* (1981), suggests several ways of getting attention for your interest in authorship. Tell published friends about your desire to write for a book. A personal introduction from them to a publishing insider is a wonderful boost to your ambition. Talk to publishers' sales representatives about your interest in or ideas for writing a book. They may be able to alert you to like-minded individuals elsewhere. Or, better yet, they may add you to the pool of modestly paid manuscript reviewers employed by the publisher to review book proposals (more on this avenue later). For the same reason, seek to meet editors, both professional editors with publishing firms and those assigned to an association-sponsored project.

And there are other possibilities. Volunteer for a conference planning committee. Doing this increases your exposure to the movers and shakers in your field, of course, with untold potential for publishing-related contacts later. More immediately, though, the opportunity to screen program proposals exposes you to the caliber of professional writing in the field, which gives you a chance to contrast your writing ability with that of your peers. You thus can judge for yourself whether your command of the intended book topic and your writing ability are better than average and hence more likely to be appealing to a publisher.

From your position on the program committee or from an appropriate involvement elsewhere in the organization, you also might recommend that a collection of some sort be developed. If the idea is accepted, you stand a good chance of working on it. Though, as noted above, a yearbook in family medicine is currently presented, undoubtedly there is room for other book publications.

Assuming, then, that you find yourself a contributor to a book, are you going to be paid for your contribution? In a word, no. Particularly when the book is sponsored by your professional organization, you can expect little more than another citation for your CV or possibly a free copy of the finished product.

Undaunted by this news and probably eager as ever to contribute your part of the book, you should find out as much as you can about the book as a whole and your part in it from the book's initiator. The following list covers the information you need.

Need-to-Know Items for Contributing Authors

Outline of the Work as a Whole
    Chapter working titles
    Topic summaries (couple lines to couple paragraphs)
    Chapter authors
    Approximate page limits per chapter
Dates
    Deadlines for best completed manuscript
    Publication date (estimate)
Credits
    Coordinator's name
    Who will be listed, and how, on title page

    Publisher
    Bylines
    Author identification form
Style Matters
    Typing requirements for manuscript
    Headings
    Table and figures
    Reference format
Permission
    Standard form available from publisher?
    If no, locate your own
Directory of Addresses, Phone Numbers
    Coordinator
    Contributors
    For manuscript submitted

When You are the Book's Initiator

As a book's initiator (on the sending end of the above list), you may be handling either the contributions of a variety of other authors or solely your own writing. Either case poses a number of similar concerns: Where do you find a publisher? How do you approach a publisher? What about the contract? Answers to these questions follow.

Finding a Publisher

You should begin searching for a publisher as soon as you start thinking about the book's content. The process, less predictable than having an article accepted or a proposal funded, should include both commercial publishers and association publishers.

Commercial publishers are organizations in business to do nothing but publish. They typically handle texts, specialized books, anthologies, and trade books. Advice to the author approaching a commercial publisher has a bit of a Catch-22 quality to it. You want to approach a publisher who already has produced titles in your area of interest, but not so many or so well received that the turf is already claimed. In publishing it is certainly true that nothing succeeds like success. Having already ventured into the market with a book on a topic similar to yours, and having enjoyed some sales with it, a publisher is likely to consider that area again. If, however, the firm already publishes the Bible on this topic (which is now in its tenth edition besides), you might not want to play the David to that Goliath.

Association publishers are what the name implies: a professional association, educational institution, or company whose main business is not publishing, yet who occasionally do publish material pertinent to their constituents, such as a proceedings of a conference it sponsors, a yearbook for members, or a specialized monograph. Besides commercial publishers, authors should consider the organizations with which they are affiliated as possible publishing sources as well.

Specifically where do you look to find names of publishers to approach? For a proposed text, check to see who has published the texts currently available at the level you plan to target: college, medical school, research community. For specialized and trade books, check to see whose treatment of similar material you like, then approach that publisher. Once you have a name or two, you should check the firm's catalog of printed and forthcoming books. (See if the acquisition department or an appropriate library has them, or call the first to request same.) The catalog will give you an even better idea than just one book alone of the niche the publisher has created for itself.

To turn up names of other publishers, two suggestions: check out *Literary Market Place* (LMP), and consider a university press. LMP, an annual directory, is the "yellow pages" for any business having to do with book publishing, from paper suppliers to distributors. The largest section of LMP lists American publishers in alphabetical order, then in categories by geographic location, field of activity (e.g., textbooks, scholarly books), and subject matter (e.g., education, health and medicine). The main entry includes the publisher's address and telephone number, names of key staff, and a short summary of the publisher's areas of interest, among many other details pertinent to those in the industry.

Association presses and university presses also are included in LMP. These smaller, less familiar publishers are not to be overlooked, however: in 1982 alone, the 67 U.S. members of the Association of American University Presses produced over 3200 titles.

Once you have compiled a list of likely publishers, including commercial and association publishers, you must prepare a convincing package marketing your ideas to the publisher. How to do that is explained next.

How To Approach a Publisher?

The first question a publisher raises about a manuscript is, Is this book worth publishing? The next is, Will it sell? From the moment you first contact a publisher then, you should make clear your reasons for believing that the answer to both is "yes."

Publishers emphatically do not want to see your entire manuscript when you first contact them about publishing it. An outline of the whole work comes first. Later, if the publisher is interested, you will be asked to provide writing samples.

Your first contact with a publisher should be a query letter, a one- to two-page letter that includes three kinds of information. First, you should give a good idea of the proposed book as a whole. A fully developed outline is not necessary in an initial query, though one eventually will be required. Next you should directly contrast your planned book with similar ones. This comparison accomplishes two purposes. It informs publishers of the competition (although if you have selected wisely, the publisher should be an appropriate one for your title and thus already abundantly aware of the competition). Stating other books on the shelves also enables the publisher to judge your knowledge of the field you are writing for, of books and of publishing. The third element of a query letter is a description of yourself and your competence to write the book you propose.

The query should be addressed to the relevant department of a publishing house and to the appropriate person. Both details are listed in *Literary Market Place*. Receipt of your query may be acknowledged; a definite response will arrive in the publisher's good time. Because the system is sluggish, an author may send queries to several publishers simultaneously. If you do this, however, you should note that fact in the query letter.

Let us assume that you have struck a responsive chord in the first editor who reads your query. A cordial letter (and carefully worded so as not to promise *anything*) will be sent to you, requesting a prospectus and possibly enclosing a form on which to provide additional information. Now you really have to show your stuff. Since the prospectus package will be examined by many more people than saw the original query (art director, managing editor, etc.), feel free to repeat materials included in the query letter.

Manuscript Reviewers

Typically in the case of specialized books and texts, besides the publishing house staff, one or more paid, outside experts will also review and comment on your prospectus. Though the stipend is modest, some authors have found this job of manuscript reviewer to be a valuable one for several reasons. Through it they have an entree into a particular publisher's decision-making process; they have a chance to demonstrate their own organizing and writing abilities by preparing critiques of the same for others; and from this vantage point, they can make a realistic appraisal of what it takes to prepare a convincing prospectus.

The prospectus should include five items:

(1) An up-to-date resume.
(2) Detailed outline with extensive subheadings.
(3) Tentative table of contents with chapter titles.
(4) One at least and preferably more sample chapters (these need not follow in chronological order from the contents).

(5) A one- to two-page cover letter summarizing highlights of the accompanying materials. Here is no place for false modesty.

Remember you are selling the worth of your ideas and your experience, so pull out all the persuasive stops!

In this success scenario, the next step is signing a publishing contract, a happy event discussed briefly below.

Signing a Book Contract

Of many points to be covered in a complete treatment of book contracts, suffice it to note the following.

Realize that the "standard" contract you are shown is only one of a half-dozen or more that the publisher routinely makes available. Thus, treat the contract as you might an initial job interview: You will want to check out the publisher in your turn. Talk to published colleagues about both the terms of their contracts and the details of their negotiating process. Discuss with an attorney anything you do not understand and especially anything you wish to change.

For further information on book contracts and book publishing in general, refer to Van Til's book mentioned above and Balkin (1977). The American Society of Journalists and Authors and the Writers' Guild also provide much useful information (you must have had one book published to be eligible for membership in the guild).

Humankind is uniquely equipped for communicating via language. And few language activities are as absorbing and rewarding as writing for publication. I hope this guidebook to the journey has whetted your interest in making the trip toward any writing destination. *Bon voyage! Bon courage!*

Faculty Development Activities

(1) Describe your goals in medical writing. How will attainment of these goals affect your career?
(2) List the medical publications most important to you and your professional colleagues.
(3) List the articles you have read in the past week or two. Evaluate one of them in regard to structure, content, and clarity. Tell the major themes of the article.
(4) Write a letter to the editor commenting on one of the articles listed in Activity 3.
(5) Tell the similarities and differences among: (1) case report, (2) literature review, and (3) book chapter. Plan an outline for one of these types of medical writing.

References

Balkin R. A writer's guide to book publishing. New York: Hawthorn Books, 1977.

Beatty WK. Searching the literature and computerized services in medicine. Ann Int Med 1979;91:326–32.

Bland CJ. Faculty development through workshops. Springfield, Illinois: Charles C Thomas, 1980.

Conn H, Rakel R, Johnson T (eds). Family practice. Philadelphia: WB Saunders, 1973.

Cooper HM. Scientific guidelines for conducting integrative research reviews. Rev Educ Res 1982;52:291–302.

Currie MN (ed). Patient education in the primary care setting: 5th annual conference. Kansas City, Missouri: St. Mary's Hospital of Kansas City Family Practice Residency, 1983.

Fabb WE, Heffernan MW, Phillips WA, Stone P. Focus on learning in family practice. Melbourne: Royal Australian College of General Practitioners, 1976.

Gehlbach SH. Interpreting the medical literature. Lexington, Massachusetts: D. C. Heath and Company, 1982.

Huth EJ. How to write and publish papers in the medical sciences. Philadelphia, ISI Press, 1982, ch 6.

Ladas H. Summarizing research: A case study. Rev Educ Res 1980;50:597–624.

Lipkin M Jr, Boufford J, Froom J, White KL (eds). Primary care research in 1981: The collected abstracts of five medical societies. New York: The Rockefeller Foundation, 1982.

Moo-Dodge MM, Bland CJ. A case for reviewing the literature. Fam Med 1981 May–June;13:20–1.

Nahum AM. The clinical case report: "Potboiler" or scientific literature? Head Neck Surg 1979;1:291 2.

Rodnick JE, Ransom DC. Standard nomenclature in presentations, letter. Fam Med 1983 Jan/Feb; 25:25.

Roland CG. Thoughts about medical writing, No. 31: The letter-to-the-editor. Anesth Analg 1975;54:626–7.

Rubin A. An unwritten "case report," letter. N Engl J Med 1979;300:96.

Soffer A. Case reports of untoward drug reactions, adverse events, and rare diseases, editorial. Arch Int Med 1982;142:1271–2.

Stoan SK. Computer searching: A primer for the uninformed scholar. Academe 1982 Nov–Dec;68:10–15.

Taylor RB (ed). Family medicine: Principles and practice, second edition. New York: Springer-Verlag, 1983.

Thorne C. Better medical writing. London: Pitman Medical and Scientific Publishing, 1970, ch 10.

Van Til W. Writing for professional publication. Boston: Allyn and Bacon, Inc., 1981.

Chapter 5

Writing for Communication with the Public

Susan Okie

Why Write for the Public?

Doctors and journalists traditionally regard one another with mutual distrust. In my experience as a physician covering medicine for the *Washington Post*, and more recently as the author of a health column for *Cosmopolitan Magazine*, I have been amply exposed to the grudges and prejudices each profession holds toward the other. Physicians frequently get the chance to observe the spats and reconciliations in this rocky relationship, when members of one camp or the other hold forth on the editorial pages of medical journals.

The same themes tend to recur. Doctors invariably complain that medical articles appearing in the popular press are inaccurate, shallow, and sensational (Barclay, 1979; Soffer, 1978). They charge that reporters ignore the caveats appended to researchers' findings, and encourage the public to expect magical cures and simple answers. They claim that the press's portrayal of the health care system paints doctors as greedy and impersonal, eroding patients' trust and converting the doctor-patient relationship into an adversarial one.

Journalists, for their part, complain that physicians are paranoid about media coverage (Grace, 1980). They often find researchers inaccessible— either unwilling to explain their findings, or worried that granting interviews may prevent their work from being published in medical journals (a consequence of the much-publicized "Ingelfinger-Relman

Rule" at the *New England Journal of Medicine*). They view doctors as patronizing in their attitude toward reporters, unwilling to believe in an interviewer's intelligence or competence. And they consider doctors overly paternalistic toward patients, reluctant to relinquish any of their autonomy over decisions that affect patient care.

Enlightened observers on both sides have often pointed out that the dearth of cooperation between medicine and the press prevents the media from being used to fullest advantage as a force for health education (Bander, 1975; DeBakey, 1981; Houston, 1982). There is abundant evidence of the impact of media coverage on public awareness of health issues: Witness the surge of reported cases of toxic-shock syndrome that followed press reports of the new illness in 1980 (Davis, 1982), or the prompt drop in sales of Tylenol after an outbreak of deaths from product-tampering in 1982.

And the public's appetite for health information and medical news is higher than ever. Reader surveys conducted by large newspapers and magazines consistently show that health is one of the areas of highest interest, and that medical columns are among the best-read features. By ignoring this hunger for information and by refusing to participate in the media's attempts to satisfy it, responsible members of the medical profession all too often abandon the field to others who use medical publicity irresponsibly and selfishly (Rourk, 1981).

One partial remedy for this situation is to have more physicians become skilled in writing for the general public. Acquiring this skill offers benefits both for the individual doctor and for the profession as a whole. Learning to explain a medical problem in simple terms makes a physician more effective in communicating with his or her own patients, both orally and through brochures and information sheets prepared for distribution in the office or clinic (Anderson, 1980; Laher, 1981). It allows the physician to extend this power to communicate by writing articles for publication in newspapers or magazines, thereby reaching a much wider audience. It renders the physician more intelligible and, thus, more likely to be quoted fairly and accurately in interviews with reporters. Finally, it imparts to the physician a deeper understanding of the constraints hampering reporters, and of the skill required to write a balanced, accurate medical article for the lay reader. Such an understanding, in the long run, would make for friendlier relations between doctors and press.

First, Know Thy Audience

The three elements to be considered in planning and writing an article (on any topic) are content, structure, and style. The article's content is the information it seeks to convey; its structure, the format chosen for presenting the information, including such considerations as total length, subdivisions, and illustrations; its style is the "voice" adopted by the author, and is created by the choice of words and the building of sentences.

Before a writer can make decisions concerning any of these three elements, he or she must consider the audience who will read the finished article. How deep is their interest in the topic to be discussed, and how can that interest be heightened? How much background knowledge can the writer assume they have? What are the factors that might prevent them from reading the article, or finishing it once they begin?

An experienced newspaper editor could teach most physicians a great deal about this subject. The interest with which most readers approach a medical article is practical: They want to know how the information affects their lives. They wish to prolong life and health and to avoid illness; they want to be informed about hazards to their well-being and about the sufferings of others, and they want to know how to escape harm themselves. These are natural feelings, and from them springs the susceptibility to promises and "cures" that is a part of human nature. This susceptibility is present in everyone—even physicians—and is a force for both good and evil in medical writing.

Coupled with the reader's desire for sound medical advice is a universal reluctance to change. Most people are creatures of habit, addicted to their high-cholesterol diets, their sedentary life-styles, and their multiple sources of stress. Most are aware that some of their habits are bad for them, but they do not like to hear it. Time after time, as a reporter, I saw overweight editors look bored and disgruntled when they read stories on the merits of jogging, only to perk up when they spotted a report of a jogger who dropped dead of a cardiac arrest. The medical writer must constantly grapple with the fact that readers are hoping to receive something for nothing, not to be told that they must relinquish a cherished habit or adopt a disagreeable one. Getting people to face the truth about their bodies requires active persuasion.

Many readers are fascinated with the technological aspects of medicine and with the workings of the human body, and will readily be attracted by vivid descriptions of an operation, a scientific discovery, or a cellular event. But most do not have a clear idea of the day-to-day work of a doctor or a scientist. Because there is little public awareness of the gradual, tentative and sometimes myopic process by which new medical knowledge is acquired and tested, readers often become impatient with the statement that "further research is needed" before a new treatment can be accepted. Some even suspect that medical experts withhold remedies from the public for reasons of their own—an attitude that unfortunately makes them vulnerable to apostles of untested "alternative therapies" for such diseases as cancer or arthritis.

Articles on medicine for the public must be written with a clear awareness of the difference between literacy and technical knowledge. The average reader, however intelligent, has not had a course in human physiology and cannot be assumed to know how the body's organ systems work. Names of some organs such as the heart, lungs, stomach, and brain are universally recognized, and their purpose is understood in a general way. The purpose of others such as the liver, kidneys, spleen, or bone marrow ought to be mentioned in a phrase or sentence whenever they are introduced. Whenever a reader's comprehension of a medical treatment or discovery requires more detailed knowledge of how an organ performs its function, the writer should pause to explain its performance in simple terms.

Words such as "lesion," "immunity," "ligate," "abscess," and "bronchi" are too technical for the average reader, and must be either explained or replaced by simpler words. The problem of judging the technical difficulty of a piece of writing has prompted the development of a number of "readability tests" in which the writer counts the number of technical or polysyllabic words contained in a piece and then performs a mathematical manipulation to arrive at the educational level required to understand it (Freimuth, 1979; Spardaro, 1980). Researchers who have applied such tests to patient consent forms or to pharmaceutical package inserts have concluded that most of these materials require at least high school, and sometimes college-level education on the part of readers (Cassileth, 1980; Morrow, 1980). When it is crucial that a piece of medical writing be understood even by someone who has had only an elementary school education, applying a "readability test" can be very helpful. For a more highly educated audience, it usually suffices for the writer to try out his or her work on friends or family members who do not have a medical background.

Apart from the educational background required to understand a medical article, there are emotional impediments to learning about the body which a writer must recognize in order to surmount. Foremost is the reader's natural denial of his own mortality—denial that expresses itself in squeamishness over the "gory" details of illness and its treatment, or in outright terror when confronted with the facts of old age, degenerative disease, and death (Thomas, 1972). Newspaper editors recognize this quality of denial when they talk about the "breakfast test": the question whether an article can safely be read while eating eggs and toast. A description that seems clinically correct to a physician may be frighteningly or nauseatingly graphic to a lay reader. The writer must balance the desire to paint a clear picture against the danger of turning off readers if the picture is too vivid.

The other "reader's block" to be mentioned is fear of scientific or technical material. Many people, because they had trouble with math or science during school, assume that they will have trouble understanding a medical article—so they refuse to try. The writer must seduce them into reading, often by deemphasizing the technical side of the story and telling it, as far as possible, from the personal viewpoint of a patient, family member, doctor, or scientist. This is especially important in choosing an opening sentence or "lede" for the story, the strongest determinant of whether the reader will read on. For example, one article I wrote for the *Washington Post* in 1980 on the topic of reconstructive facial surgery (Okie, 1980 Aug.) opened by describing the emotional plight of a young man with a facial deformity, whose schoolmates had always called him "Frankenstein." The description of his operation began lower in the article, and was divided into sections that alternated with a discussion of his family, his self-image, and his reasons for having surgery that would transform him. In this way, the reluctance that a reader might feel about visualizing the complicated, "gory" operation could be overcome by sympathy for the patient.

Content

The range of material available and appropriate for medical articles is as vast as medicine itself. One need only consider the spectrum of topics treated by such writers as Lewis Thomas, Burton Roueché, and Daniel S. Greenberg, all three of whom write about medicine for the general public. Most individual newspapers or magazines, however, cover only a small portion of the available ground. For instance, a 1981 study by the Proudfoots of medical articles in Australian newspapers found that 33% dealt with warnings or reports of adverse reactions, 27% with "new" discoveries (not always truly new), 12% with criticism of health care personnel and institutions, and 6% with advice about health maintenance. The proportions in other newspapers might vary, but the categories are probably representative.

Family physicians would probably be most interested in the category of "advice on health maintenance." Editors are usually eager for such articles, which they consider both consumer-oriented and convenient, since they usually need not run on a particular day or week but can be fitted in as space allows. Some seasonal articles are so perennially popular that, seeing them, I suffer the same reaction as on seeing the first robin of spring: A story on head lice in school children means it is fall, a story on influenza means it is winter, a story on hangovers means it is New Year's Day or Eve. Others are appropriate at any time of year, such as articles on health screening (how often to have a physical, Pap smear, mammogram), common disorders (high blood pressure, breast cancer, ulcers, ear infections) or prevention (smoking, exercise, alcohol, seatbelts, and infant seats). Despite the relevance of such topics, editors will often be more eager to run them if they are somehow tied to recent events. For instance, an article on physical examinations and screening might be welcome when presidential candidates had just released their medical reports, or an article on immunizations would be well received just after a local case of polio had been reported.

Stories warning of risks to the community's health are of paramount importance, and will generally be given top priority by newspapers. A physician can often serve as the source or instigator of such a story, on or off the record, even if he or she does not feel qualified to write it. For instance, pediatricians in Washington D.C. provided the initial impetus for articles published in the *Post* in 1979 on a defective infant formula (Okie, 1979 Oct.), and in the same year a physician newly appointed to head the city's tuberculosis program gave me the information needed to report on Washington's failure to stem that disease among its poor (Okie, 1979 Nov.).

News stories by doctors evaluating the quality of care in a community are likely to be viewed with suspicion by editors, because of the possibility of bias or conflict of interest. However, it may at times be appropriate for a physician to write such an article—perhaps as an op-ed (opinion-editorial) piece—especially if he or she has special expertise from serving on a local commission or hospital committee. Often, physicians are moved to rebut a publication's criticisms of local institutions or medical practices, either by writing an op-ed article or by giving an interview. If the writer's intention is to answer criticism, an angry, defensive tone will be far less effective than a calm, logical, point-by-point reply.

One much-neglected side of medical reporting is the day-to-day experience of medical practice or research: its rewards, its frustrations, its constraints (Greenberg, 1977). Physicians could do much to counter charges of impersonality and greed in the American health care system by writing a personal account of a busy day in a city hospital or a rural family practice. Issues involving Medicaid, health insurance, nursing home care, diagnostic tests, and patient education could all be made clearer and more interesting in this kind of format. Similarly, an account by a scientist or clinical investigator of, for example, the tribulations of conducting a clinical trial or a chart review would give readers new insight into what researchers mean when they qualify a discovery by saying "further studies are needed."

Structure

The typical news story published by a newspaper on a medical topic measures 12 to 18 "column-inches," perhaps 400 to 700 words. An op-ed piece or a "take-out" (the slang term for a definitive, detailed story) is longer—up to four or five times the length of an average news story. A magazine article on a medical subject may be longer still, while a "short," frequently condensed from a wire-service story and inserted in a newspaper to fill space may be only one or two paragraphs long.

Regardless of length, all such articles begin with a "lede," an opening sentence or short paragraph that usually states the point of the story, combines some of the critical facts (who, what, when, where, why), and—if successful—captures the reader's attention. In working with reporters on articles, editors devote most of their time and attention to the lede, for two reasons. First, they know that the first few sentences of a news story determine whether the reader reads farther. And second, the facts and assertions in the first few sentences, and the order in which they are presented, often provide an automatic structure for the rest of the article (Webb, 1978).

Most newspaper stories begin with a "hard-news" lede, a one-sentence summary of the information in the article. The following are "hard-news" ledes for imaginary stories:

> Interferon has proven dramatically effective in combating virus infections in cancer patients, according to research reported yesterday by Yale University physicians.

> Local health authorities warned yesterday that measles is making a comeback among toddlers in the city's day-care centers.

The lede for a "take-out" or a consumer-oriented article, written to provide information but not tied to a particular event, may contain fewer particulars of time and place but still summarizes the point of the story. For example,

> Auto accidents and heat exhaustion are the two most serious hazards to joggers, but both are usually avoidable if the runner takes a few simple precautions.

Finally, a feature story, magazine article, and even some news stories may utilize a "soft" or anecdotal lede, which piques the reader's interest without immediately revealing the thrust of the article. This is one of the "seduction" techniques described earlier, by which the reader can be drawn into the personal situation of a character in the story before he or she realizes that the article is about science or medicine. For example,

> Anne remembers vividly the day her leukemia was diagnosed. It was the day she came to the hospital to give birth to her daughter.

After reading this lede, the reader would realize that the article dealt with leukemia, but he or she would not know whether it would discuss new treatments for the disease, the shock of learning the diagnosis, Anne's and her family's experiences, or some other aspect of the illness. In contrast, the news ledes presented earlier contain everything the reader needs to guess what will follow.

In newspapers, the opening few paragraphs of a story are usually no more than one or two sentences long. Although the rules of style for essays and fiction forbid treating single sentences as paragraphs (except when the sentence serves as a transition), newspaper style commonly does so. This is because, when set in columns, a paragraph of average length becomes visually unwieldly and difficult to read. One- or two-sentence paragraphs are much easier on the reader's eyes. They are the building blocks of most newspaper articles. In a magazine, depending on the printing style and the length of each printed line, paragraphs can be somewhat longer.

The paragraphs immediately following the lede should give additional important facts and should provide a broader context for the story. Editors often refer to the second or third paragraph of an article as the "so-what 'graph," because it answers the reader's mental question, "So what?" In other words, it explains why the news reported in the lede is significant, if the lede itself has not already done so.

Here is an example from a 1980 article that I wrote for the *Washington Post* (Okie, 1980 June):

Lede:

> The use of tampons has been linked to a mysterious and sometimes fatal new disease that most often strikes women under 30, federal disease investigators said yesterday.

Additional details:

> The new clue to the cause of toxic-shock syndrome, which occurs during or just after the patient's menstrual period, was reported by investigators for the Center for Disease Control in Atlanta.

So-what paragraph:

> New reports of the illness have been mounting rapidly at the center since it published a bulletin May 23 on the disease. Since September 1978, there have been 131 reported cases of toxic-shock syndrome, 10 of them fatal. All but three of the victims were women, including the 10 who died. (Reprinted with permission from the Washington Post, June 28, 1980, p. 1).

In this example, the research discovery reported in the lede receives added significance from the so-what paragraph, which provides figures on the disease outbreak and the number of deaths. In medical stories, the so-what paragraph typically contains information on the incidence of a disease or treatment or the cost to society. For instance, a 1981 article on childhood ear infections (Okie, 1981) opened with a prevalence figure (70% of American children) and raised questions about the infections' potential effects on hearing, speech, and intellectual development. The second paragraph (a so-what paragraph) gave figures for the number of visits to the doctor prompted by ear infections each year, and the annual cost. The third paragraph (another so-what paragraph) reported the growing number of myringotomies being done annually for insertion of tubes to drain middle-ear effusions. The fourth introduced a secondary lede, the growing controversy over the need for such surgery.

It should be clear from these two examples that, once the lede and the so-what paragraphs are in place, much of the content and sequence of the succeeding paragraphs will logically follow. In the article on toxic-shock syndrome, the next few paragraphs briefly explained the syndrome's suspected bacterial etiology and the epidemiologic characteristics of its victims. A summary of the evidence for its connection with tampons followed, coupled with the CDC's recommendations to tampon users. Next came the investigators' qualifications of their findings, and comments from tampon manufacturers. The final paragraphs of the story described the symptoms of toxic-shock syndrome (material that had been reported in previous articles) and advised readers about its diagnosis and treatment.

In deciding the order of the facts reported in the body of a medical article, the writer should consider carefully what implications the information will have for readers, and how a reader's grasp of the point of the story will be affected if he or she does not read the entire piece. If warnings or advice are being offered, they should appear near the beginning and sometimes should be highlighted by boldface type, "bullets" (boldface dots placed at the beginnings of crucial paragraphs), or a separate box that accompanies the main story and repeats the important advice. If a study's authors or other investigators in the field have made comments that place a research finding in context for the reader, those comments should appear high in the story, not close to the end. If an article is sharply critical of a person, institution, or product, comments from those being criticized must be sought, and should follow either the initial statement of criticism or the evidence supporting the criticism, or both.

When reporting the findings of a study, the writer should describe the study's design, including the number of subjects, duration of the study, and results. It is not necessary to provide all the data and "p" values, since general readers will not be able to interpret such information and expert readers will want to look up the study for themselves. Instead, the writer should make efforts to determine the study's significance—by exercising his or her own expertise or by consulting others in the field—and should include comments by researchers on the importance of the findings.

If an article follows a "feature" format, describing a patient's treatment or a day in the life of a surgeon, it will depart from the structure described for a typical news article, but it will still contain some of the same components. So-what paragraphs should still appear early in the story, explaining its relevance—the seriousness of the disease, the effectiveness of a new treatment, the importance of the doctor's work. Although a chronological account of the subject's experience will be the backbone of the story, the writer must insert paragraphs where appropriate explaining pathophysiology, hospital procedure, standard treatments, or whatever else the reader needs to understand the article. It takes considerable planning and skill to weave such information into the piece without departing for long from the individual who is the focus of the reader's interest.

One other possible format for a medical article, inappropriate for newspaper use but popular for patient brochures and public-relations "fact sheets," is the question-and-answer format. In this simple structural device, the writer poses a series of questions about a topic one by one, and and answers each in a paragraph or two. The choice of questions and the order in which they are asked and answered are determined by their potential interest for the reader and, as in a news article, by which facts the writer considers most important. For instance, an article or brochure on genital herpes infections might begin with questions like, "How many Americans have herpes?" and "How does a person get a herpes infection?" and then might proceed to questions like, "What should I do if I develop herpes sores?" "How contagious is the disease?" and "What are the chances that it can be cured?"

The question-and-answer format is easy to use, and is practical for the reader because he or she can quickly find the sections of the article that are of greatest interest. This format is, of course, the standard one for "Dear Doctor" columns which reply to readers' letters. The device's chief disadvantage is that readers will skip questions that do not immediately strike them as personally relevant. This is no problem if the format is being used in a brochure that a patient will keep for future reference, but it detracts from the educational impact of the article if it is likely to be read only once and discarded.

Style

"There is no satisfactory explanation of style, no infallible guide to good writing, no assurance that a person who thinks clearly will be able to write clearly, no key that unlocks the door, no inflexible rule by which the young writer may shape his course." So wrote E. B. White, that master of style, in the chapter he added to *The Elements of Style* by William Strunk, Jr., when the Macmillan Company reissued the book in 1959. There may be no infallible guide to good writing, but Strunk and White's small gem *The Elements of Style*, reprinted many times since then, comes as close as any book can.

Strunk and White's advice on how to choose words, build sentences, and order paragraphs applies to every kind of writing, and is an invaluable starting point for the would-be medical writer. Others have written primers specifically for authors of medical articles (Gray, 1982; Manning,

1981). Some of the pointers they contain apply to all good writing; others apply particularly to technical material, and have been mentioned earlier in the section on knowing one's audience. I recommend the article "Writing Readable Health Messages" by Diane Manning, listed in the bibliography at the end of this chapter. Among her suggestions, I concur heartily with the following:

Write in the active voice.

Write short sentences containing one idea.

Place the main idea at the beginning of each paragraph.

Do not overuse connectives ("therefore," "however," "nevertheless," and similar words).

Define difficult words, and provide phonetic pronunciation when appropriate.

Use open space, subtitles, short paragraphs, and other devices to break up the narrative. (It is less taxing for the reader.)

Make the story as personal as possible, by describing individuals, using quotations, or inserting humor.

The easiest way for me to illustrate the kind of choices that determine style is to present, sentence by sentence, portions of a column on influenza vaccination written in 1982 by a fellow resident, Dr. Jeffrey Hanson, for one of Hartford's community newspapers, the *Hill Ink*. I edited Dr. Hanson's rough draft, and he then revised the article. The following examples (reprinted by permission) are sentences from the draft with my suggested revisions and the reasons for them.

Lede:

> It may seem premature to think about the 1982–83 influenza season while summer is still in session, but the U.S. Public Health Service through its Advisory Committee on Immunization Practices has just released the information on this year's vaccine.

This lede is too long and is weighed down by the title of a government agency which means nothing to the reader and delays the punch line.

Revised lede:

> It may seem premature to think about this winter's flu season, but this year's flu vaccine is now available and it's time to consider getting a "flu shot."

This lede gets right to the point, and uses the colloquial term "flu," which is familiar to the reader.

Dr. Hanson's draft continued:

> Influenza is a viral disease that affects the respiratory tract. Infection with the virus can cause anything from mild upper respiratory tract symptoms with fever, malaise, and muscular pain to pneumonia. Certain identifiable groups of people are at higher risk for a serious influenzal infection or even death. These include children and adults with chronic lung or heart disease as well as anyone who is immunocompromised (transplant and cancer patients).

The article proceeds logically by defining influenza and identifying those to whom it poses the greatest threat. But it is full of technical and unnecessary words. My suggested revision:

> Influenza, or 'flu,' is caused by a virus that attacks the lungs and air passages. Infection with the virus can cause symptoms ranging from sore throat and congestion with fever and muscle aches to pneumonia. Certain people are at higher risk for a serious or even fatal influenza infection. These include children and adults with chronic lung or heart disease, or anyone whose natural defenses against illness are weakened (such as patients with cancer, kidney failure, or organ transplants).

Before changing its tack, a public-service article of this type should, at this point, set forth a complete summary of the groups who should receive the vaccine, state how often they need it, and mention any contraindications (in this case, egg allergy). This will ensure that readers who stop reading before they finish the article will absorb the main points.

The article went on to describe how the campaign to develop a long-lasting influenza vaccine has been hampered by the virus's ability to change each year through genetic mutations. It explained how major epidemics have occurred each time the virus undergoes a major mutation. The next paragraph read:

> The government must try to predict what variety of the influenza virus will be prominent each winter and prepare the appropriate vaccine anew each year. The result of this is a different vaccine each year that must be offered to high-risk patients and is yet only 75 to 85 percent effective.

These sentences repeat the words "vaccine" and "each" too many times. The sentences are too long, and are awkwardly strung together by "ands." The second sentence begins with one idea, then abruptly introduces a second, unrelated one. A suggested revision:

> Government scientists try each year to predict what variety of influenza virus will predominate the following winter. They prepare a new vaccine every summer, which doctors then offer to high-risk patients. The vaccine does not confer total protection, since up to 25% of recipients still contract the illness if they are exposed to the virus. But for members of high-risk groups, a yearly 'flu shot' is an important safeguard.

The only way to achieve excellent style is to write and rewrite, preferably with the assistance of a talented editor. The writer should be ruthless with his or her own copy, rereading it over and over to prune out unnecessary words, to replace technical ones, and to break up unwieldy sentences and paragraphs. When I completed the draft of my first article for the *Washington Post* in 1975, I proudly showed it to an experienced science reporter. He took a thick pencil and crossed out every other word. Then he handed it back to me to read. It still made sense.

Faculty Development Activities

(1) Review local and/or national newspapers and magazines for medical/health related articles and columns. What did you like or dislike about the various articles as regards both content and style?
(2) Invite a local newspaper reporter to a faculty meeting. Ask him/her to describe the process he/she uses to gather information and write an article for the public. If there has been a health related article you have particularly liked, you might focus discussion on that article.
(3) Invite a local newspaper editor and/or TV newsperson and discuss the following:
   - When and how to use medical language with the public?
   - What does the public request or like to read about health/medicine?
   - How to write patient education and/or clinical practice marketing materials.
(4) Pick a topic for a medical article for the newspaper. Outline the content from your perspective. Then ask several patients or non-medical friends what they would like to know about the topic. Compare the perspectives.
(5) Compare the differences in content and style between writing for commercial publications with writing for scientific publications.

References

Anderson JE, Morrell DC, Avery AJ, Watkins CJ. Evaluation of a patient education manual. Br Med J 1980;281:924–6.

Bander MS. The physician and the press. N Engl J Med 1975;293:402–3.

Barclay WR. Science reporting to alarm the public. J Am Med Assoc 1979; 242:754.

Cassileth BR, et al. Informed consent—why are its goals imperfectly realized? N Engl J Med 1980;302:896–900.

Davis JP, Vergeront JM. The effect of publicity on the reporting of toxic-shock syndrome in Wisconsin. J Inf Dis 1982;145:449–57.

DeBakey L, DeBakey S. Journal editors and the press: cooperation not conflict (letter). J Am Med Assoc 1981;245:2296–7.

Freimuth VS. Assessing the readability of health education messages. Public Health Rep 1979;94:568–70.

Grace J. Bridging the gap between medicine and the media. Can Med Assoc J 1980;122:450–2.

Gray JAM. Preparing a leaflet for patient education. Br Med J 1982;284:1171–2.

Greenberg DS. The press and health care. N Engl J Med 1977;297:231–2.

Houston TP. Alternatives in patient education: using the commercial media (letter). N Engl J Med 1982;306:998.

Laher M, et al. Educational value of printed information for patients with hypertension. Br Med J 1981;282:1360–1.

Manning D. Writing readable health messages. Public Health Rep 1981;96:464–5.

Morrow GR. How readable are subject consent forms? J Am Med Assoc 1980;244:56–8.

Okie S. A second opinion on children's ear surgery. Washington Post 1981 May 27:C1.

Okie S. Dangerous formula. Washington Post 1979 Oct. 10:A1.

Okie S. Mystery disease in women tied to tampon use. Washington Post 1980 June 28:A1.

Okie S. 'Runaway' TB in District: a public health failure. Washington Post 1979 Nov. 24:A1.

Okie S. Surgeon rebuilds a face—and a life. Washington Post 1980 Aug. 31:A1.

Proudfoot AD, Proudfoot J. Medical reporting in the lay press. Med J Australia 1981;1:8–9.

Rourk MH, Hock RA, Pursell JS, Jones D, Spock A. The news media and the doctor-patient relationship. N Engl J Med 1981;305:1278–80.

Soffer A. Patient education versus irresponsible journalism. Heart Lung 1978; 7:245–6.

Spadaro DC, Robinson LA, Smith LT. Assessing readability of patient information materials. Am J Hosp Pharm 1980;37:215–21.

Strunk WS, White EB. The elements of style. New York: Macmillan, 1959.

Thomas L. The long habit. N Engl J Med 1972; 286:825–6.

Webb RA (ed.) The Washington Post deskbook on style. New York: McGraw-Hill, 1978.

Part III

Administrative Communication

Chapter 6

Administrative Communication by Written Correspondence

E. P. Donatelle

Introduction

The purpose of this chapter is to highlight those characteristics of written administrative communication that distinguish it from other forms of writing. Understanding the basic fundamentals of good writing represents only a part of all that is required for effectively transmitting a message accurately, clearly, and appropriately. Fundamentals used as a guide to writing will be described. But more important, the use of these basic rules will be discussed within the context of a systematic "inventory" approach as to how we can improve administrative written communicative skills. Styles used in certain situations will be discussed, and finally the mechanics of using certain communication instruments will be demonstrated.

Billions of dollars are spent yearly in business, industry, and educational institutions on written forms of communication. Yet little thinking and effort are expended in *improving* the effectiveness of administrative writing. There are several reasons for this disparity.

Somehow, there is a mistaken notion that basic fundamentals of writing, if strictly adhered to, serve equally well in all writing situations. This thought is implied in the question frequently heard in discussions of writing, "What is so different about administrative writing?"

During the last two decades, the widespread use of advanced methods of communication such as the telephone, audio-video tapes, new televideo communication systems with computer storing capability, and word processors has given some persons the incorrect impression that written communication is archaic and will rapidly become "a thing of the past."

And finally, little emphasis is being given in educational institutions as to the value of the skill and art involved in administrative writing. In this regard, topics concerning administrative written communication are increasingly being added to curricula in faculty development and administrative enrichment programs.

The historian, scholar, scientist, educator, artist, businessman, and news reporter all find writing necessary for success and have developed specific models for its use. So too, administrative communication by written correspondence deserves special attention to meet the specific objectives necessary in business and medical administration.

Administrative writings are mainly for the purpose of communication among faculty, employees, and related public. It is important for the reader to understand the subtle, but real difference between *communicating* and *communication*. The simplest definition of *communicate* (Webster Unabridged Dictionary) is the following: A verb defined to mean, to make another or others partakers of: impart, transmit as news, a disease, or an idea. However, *communication* is a noun which defines the act of communicating: intercourse, exchange of ideas, conveyance of information as in correspondence. Communication is a dynamic process by which a writer documents an item that is to be communicated to which there is an anticipated tacit, emotional, or physical response. This is unlike the verbal messages presented by radio, TV, or similar modality which are heard and viewed, but do not serve the purpose of communication unless responded to by individuals concerned. Thus, administrative communication by written correspondence takes on a true meaning of personal interaction and is unlike many other writings such as found in medical literature or novels, in which the author may not necessarily anticipate nor be interested in the reader's response.

The skill and art involved in a written letter or memorandum are more than what you say; it is how you say it. As stated by Fielden (1982), "Your message, your real intentions, can get lost in your words." Viewing the entire message a communication can convey is more than understanding the dictionary's definition of the words you choose. It is also discerning the intentions, the emphases, and the relationships reflected in the connotations of those words and the sentence structures you use. Writing an effective letter is far more than stating the basic message you wish to give to someone. It is also conveying how you wish to relate to the recipient, and what you want that person to feel in response—which is important because it may determine what the reader does about the message.

One of the purposes of written communication is persuasion (Moore, 1962). It becomes a strategy of power, a model of building friendships and influencing people. Its antithesis is misunderstanding or ignorance of the communicated message which gives rise to improper attitudes and values. There is a certain charisma one either possesses or must learn as a writer. Those able to achieve this quality often become leaders in both business and educational fields. Thus in administration, especially where it involves a select group of highly motivated persons as is true in medical educational institutions, written communications must be done in a fashion that presents a message accurately, clearly, and appropriately—for total understanding without intimidation or alienation of the reader—and allowing for a reasoned, informed reponse.

"The ability to communicate" is generally accepted as a prime requisite for success in any field (Randle, 1956). And in all aspects of communication, the written form is the most troublesome. Not only does the formal nature of the message usually presented in the form of a cold paper or document pose a problem, but also the communicator is denied the benefit of tone of voice, facial expression, and gesture to aid communication. One cannot sense the reader's reaction. The message is "the record" which, for the moment, cannot be undone. Further, there is often a reason for documentation in the first place, i.e., "subject is considered too crucial or significant to be entrusted to the casual short-lived verbal form" (Fielden, 1964).

The ability to write is a highly valued asset in top business and administrative posts. Young administrators soon realize that as they rise in their respective positions, they will have to supervise the writings of their subordinates. Many memos, reports, and letters written by subordinates will go out over their signature, or be passed on to others in the institution or company, and thus reflect on the caliber of the work done under their supervision (Fielden, 1982).

As a final word of introduction, word processing techniques will not make administrative tasks less dependent on words. For while the advances in this field are fine for hundreds of tabular and computer tasks, what is entered in is what comes out. And someone must write up an eventual analysis of the findings in the common language understandable by the educated reader.

Fundamental Principles of Written Communication

Successful written communication by correspondence is not the product of inspiration nor merely the spoken words set in print, but is primarily the result of knowing how to translate ideas onto paper to convey a message. To ensure success in a written project, it is best to follow a format that will ensure that all factors involved are considered. Whether the message is a memo, letter, a proposal or report, it is well to divide the writing process into five major steps (Brusaw et al., 1976). Initially, these steps must be consciously adhered to; later with practice, each of these processes become almost automatic. The ease with which one acquires these skills is directly proportional to the care used in following a systematic approach.

Five Steps to Successful Administrative Correspondence

Step 1: Preparation

Preparation for writing consists of (1) *establishing your objective*, (2) *identifying your reader* and, (3) *determining the scope of your coverage*. The establishment of an objective for the message is simply determining what you want your reader to know or be able to do when he has finished reading your letter, memo, or report. Care must be taken to be precise. A broad and/or general objective is confusing and frequently useless. An objective such as "to report on geriatric undergraduate education in U.S. medical schools" is far too broad. But "listing schools which have a defined undergraduate curriculum for teaching geriatric medicine" gives clear direction to the reader.

One must next identify the reader as precisely as possible. Is the letter to be sent to an individual or a group of individuals composed of mixed faculty and/or ancillary personnel? What does your reader already know about the subject? What are your reader's needs in regard to terminology, definitions, and basic knowledge to understand your correspondence? What about the level of education or education potential that you must speak to? If several readers are involved, one must be careful that the message does not reflect a lecturing tone (as if addressing a group rather than an individual) which may intimidate the reader. Here, it is best to consider your total audience as an individual and address your correspondence to one person. How does one assess an audience?

Assessing the Audience

Consider the following in planning your approach to the audience:

I. Composition of the Audience
   A. Size (large group, small group, multiple readers)
   B. Kind of people
   C. Level of experience
   D. Level of education
   E. Prior knowledge of topic

II. Attitude of the Audience
   A. Toward the topic. How is the audience predisposed to view the topic? Is that attitude known? Can it be discovered?
   B. Toward the author. What is the audience's view of the author? What attitude does the author wish to create?

III. Stylistic Choices (After you know I and II, consider the following):
   A. Level of seriousness. From light to grave, happy to sad, informal to formal.
   B. Level of complexity. In both diction and syntax, the writer must choose between simple words in simple sentences and complex words in sophisticated sentences. Should the writer use technical words or common words? Symbols? Numbers?
   C. Level of familiarity. The writer must choose the relationship to establish with the audience. For example, should the writer sound authoritarian? Reasonable? Doubtful or uncertain? Expert?

Remember—the writer creates a relationship with the audience—be conscious of the relationship you are creating.

Determination of your objective and an identification of your audience will help you decide what to include and what not include in your writing. When you have distinguished the important from the unimportant, you have established the "scope" of your writing project. It is very important to clearly define the scope before beginning your research, the next step, or needless hours will be spent not knowing the kind and the amount of information needed to achieve your objective.

Step 2: Research

Most administrative correspondence is for the purpose of explaining something even though the communication frequently involves memos of direction, letters of gratitude, legislative interaction, peer communication, and so forth. To be effective, this kind of writing must be based on careful investigation (research) of the subject involved. The best way to accomplish this task is to compile a complete set of notes and then develop a working outline from those notes. The sources of this information can be personal interviews, questionnaires, or prior communication with the involved individuals. Of course, the amount of research that one needs depends on the project and "research" may amount to nothing more than jotting down all of your ideas before you begin to organize them.

Step 3: Organization

Material collected during the research process should be "organized" in a sequence that sorts out your ideas. Well-organized subject matter keeps the writer under control and allows the reader a means of following the writer's presentation. For example, if you were directing an individual in the use of a piece of laboratory equipment or a teaching protocol, you naturally would present the steps in the order of their occurrence. This is the "sequential method of development." A historical dissertation of an event describes "the chronological method of development." There are many other methods of development available to a writer, including spatial, increasing or decreasing order of importance, comparison, analysis, general to specific, specific to general, and cause and effect. As the writer, you must choose the method of development that best suits your subject, your reader, and your objective.

You are now ready to prepare an "outline." This process reduces large or complex subjects into manageable parts and ensures that your writing will move from idea to idea in a logical manner without omitting anything important. It also enables you to emphasize key points by placing them in positions of greatest importance. The use of an outline forces you to structure your thinking while allowing you to concentrate on writing when you begin the rough draft. Even if the task is only a letter or short memo, successful administrative writing needs the logic and structure that an outline provides. Simpler projects, after some experience, can be developed and outlined mentally rather than setting them in writing.

Step 4: Writing the Draft

The previously described steps should make the writing of a draft relatively easy. Writing the draft is simply the process of expanding the notes from your outline into topic sentences and then into paragraphs. It is well at this time to concentrate on ideas, and not be concerned with syntax, grammar, or spelling. Also many authors defer composition of introductory statements until later, and instead focus on the reader's needs.

Step 5: Revision

In this step, the writer must read and evaluate the draft from the reader's viewpoint. He must be anxious to find and correct faults, which may require that the rough draft be reviewed several times. It must be checked for accuracy and completeness. Remember that unnecessary information and loosely related topics may confuse the reader.

It is now time to think carefully of your introductory remarks, which should serve as a frame into which your reader can fit the information in the body of your correspondence. Such remarks should suggest the subject and capture the reader's attention. Your draft should have unity, coherence, and appropriate transition. All sentences in each paragraph contribute to the development of the paragraph's central idea. This is best accomplished by expressing the central ideas as a *"topic sentence."* In a sequential manner, all paragraphs should contribute to the development of the main topic.

If your paper has good coherence, the sentences and paragraphs will flow smoothly from one into the next; the relationship of each sentence or paragraph to the one before is clear. This is achieved by using transitional devices and by maintaining a consistent point of view. Careful attention should be placed on proper emphasis and subordination of your thoughts.

It is at this time that one needs to adjust the pace of the written material. If an area has too many ideas jammed together, space the ideas out and slow the pace; conversely, if you find a series of simple ideas expressed in short, choppy sentences, combine them into longer, more complex sentences.

Your draft must be checked for clarity and for freedom from affectation. The use of jargon must be consistent with your audience's understanding. A search must be made for abstract words that can be replaced by concrete words.

The following checklist by Milton Hall (1950) will help the inexperienced writer:

> Can you answer "yes" to the following questions about each piece you write? Is it: (1) *Complete?*—Does it give all necessary information; Answer all questions the reader may raise? (2) *Concise?*—Does it contain only essential facts, words and phrases? (3) *Clear?*—Is the language adapted to the reader?; Are the words the simplest that carry and express the thought?; Is the sentence structure clear?; Does a paragraph express one main idea?; Are the ideas in the best order? (4) *Correct?*—Is the information accurate, conform with policy?; Is the grammar, spelling and punctuation correct? (5) *Appropriate In Tone?*—Will the tone bring the desired response?; Is the writing free from words that may arouse antagonism?; Is it free of stilted, hackneyed or legalistic phrases? (6) *Effective?*—Does it thoroughly and directly get your message across to the reader?

Style, which will be discussed in greater detail later in the chapter, is a very important factor in administrative communication. Conciseness is an attribute of few writers and is usually learned with great difficulty. Get rid of clichés and other trite language. Although there is a great temptation to use the passive voice in administrative writing, an active voice is far stronger and also more concise.

Until one has become an experienced communicator, it is well to examine the sentence structure carefully and look for ways to achieve more interesting sentence variety. The use of a thesaurus to select synonyms often relieves boredom for the reader.

Initially, your draft will appear awkward and may appear to depart from the appropriate tone. Although "awkward" and "tone" are hard to define because they relate to a great many different things, one can obtain a sense of these two elements by reading the draft aloud or by having someone read it to you while you are listening as if you were the reader. In this manner, clumsiness will become apparent to both the reader and yourself. Be cautious of using phrases and statements that sound like lecturing. It is best to avoid trying to be witty. Correcting the tone is frequently a matter of replacing one word with another that has the appropriate connotations. For example, consider the difference in the tone between, "I am confused

Table 6-1. Written Performance Inventory*

1. Readibility

Reader's level
- ☐ Too specialized in approach
- ☐ Assumes too great a knowledge of subject
- ☐ So underestimates the reader that it belabors the obvious

Sentence construction
- ☐ Unnecessarily long in difficult material
- ☐ Subject–verb–object word order too rarely used
- ☐ Choppy, overly simple style (in simple material)

Paragraph construction
- ☐ Lack of topic sentence
- ☐ Too many ideas in single paragraph
- ☐ Too long

Familiarity of words
- ☐ Inappropriate jargon
- ☐ Pretentious language
- ☐ Unnecessarily abstract

Reader Direction
- ☐ Lack of "framing" (i.e., failure to tell the reader about purpose and direction of forthcoming discussion)
- ☐ Inadequate transitions between paragraphs
- ☐ Absence of subconclusions to summarize reader's progress at end of divisions in the discussion

Focus
- ☐ Unclear as to subject of communication
- ☐ Unclear as to purpose of message

2. Correctness

Mechanics
- ☐ Shaky grammar
- ☐ Faulty punctuation

Format
- ☐ Careless appearance of documents
- ☐ Failure to use accepted company form

Coherence
- ☐ Sentences seem awkward owing to illogical and ungrammatical yoking of unrelated ideas
- ☐ Failure to develop a logical progression of ideas through coherent, logically juxtaposed paragraphs

3. Appropriateness

A. Upward communications

Tact
- ☐ Failure to recognize differences in position between writer and receiver
- ☐ Impolitic tone—too brusk, argumentative, or insulting

Table 6.1 *(continued)*

Supporting Detail
☐ Inadequate support for statements
☐ Too much undigested detail for busy superior

Opinion
☐ Adequate research but too great an intrusion of opinions
☐ Too few facts (and too little research) to entitle drawing of conclusions
☐ Presence of unasked for but clearly implied recommendations

Attitude
☐ Too obvious a desire to please superior
☐ Too defensive in face of authority

B. Downward communications

Diplomacy
☐ Overbearing attitude toward subordinates
☐ Insulting and/or personal references
☐ Unmindfulness that messages are representative of management group or even of company

Clarification of desires
☐ Confused, vague instructions
☐ Superior is not sure of what is wanted
☐ Withholding of information necessary to job at hand

Motivational aspects
☐ Orders of superior seem arbitrary
☐ Superior's communications are manipulative and seemingly insincere

4. Thought

Preparation
☐ Inadequate thought given to purpose of communication prior to its final completion
☐ Inadequate preparation or use of data known to be available

Competence
☐ Subject beyond intellectual capabilities of writer
☐ Subject beyond experience of writer

Fidelity to assignment
☐ Failure to stick to job assigned
☐ Too much of routine assignment
☐ Too little made of assignment

Analysis
☐ Superifical examination of data leading to unconscious overlooking of important pieces of evidence
☐ Failure to draw obvious conclusions from data presented
☐ Presentation of conclusions unjustified by evidence
☐ Failure to qualify tenuous assertions
☐ Failure to identify and justify assumptions used
☐ Bias, conscious or unconscious, which leads to distorted interpretation of data

Table 6.1 *(continued)*

Persuasiveness
□ Seems more convincing than facts warrant
□ Seems less convincing than facts warrant
□ Too obvious an attempt to sell ideas
□ Lacks action-orientation and managerial viewpoint
□ Too blunt an approach where subtlety and finesse called for

---

*Reprinted by permission of the Harvard Business Review, an exhibit from "What Do You Mean I Can't Write?" by John S. Fielden (May/June 1964). Copyright © 1964 by the President and Fellows of Harvard College; all rights reserved.

by your *stubbornness* in opposing the plan" and "I am puzzled by the *firmness* of your opposition to the plan."

And finally, check slowly and carefully for problems of grammar, punctuation, mechanics (spelling, abbreviations, capital letters, etc.), and format.

If you have prepared well, considering your objective for writing, your reader, and the scope of your subject; if your research has been adequate, your outline to the point, and your paper well drafted and revised, then your correspondence will have achieved the following objectives:

(1) Stated clearly what you have wanted to say. The reader will understand your message. Remember, the message must be clear to the reader.
(2) Avoided using long verbs when a shorter one will do.
(3) Avoided using nouns to modify other nouns. You will have allowed verbs to do the work.
(4) Used the active voice whenever possible.
(5) Have kept your sentences reasonably short; complex sentences can be understood, but elaborate long sentences are difficult to comprehend.

Written Performance Inventory

Rarely is the cause of poor writing due to poor spelling, punctuation, or grammar. A failure of the ability to think and organize one's thoughts may result in a report or letter being completely unreadable. Occasionally, tactlessness, failure to sense the human relations aspect of communications, builds resentment and resistance to what has been written. The frequently nonperceived talking "down" or talking "over the head of one's readers" presents problems in effectively communicating a message. "What are the components of good writing? And, in which of these elements am I proficient? In which do I fail?" If these questions could be answered, then one could set about the task of doing something about them. Good administrative writing is not just grammar, clear thinking, or winning friends and influencing people. It is some of each, the proportion depending on the purpose.

Fielden (1964) has designed a "total inventory" protocol that can assist in determining and correcting "administrative writing deficiencies" (see Table 6-1). The use of the "Written Performance Inventory" will:

Assist top administrators in training their people to tackle problems covering administrative writing.

Impress upon persons writing the different tactics and style that must be used because of the position and power of the person being written to.

Serve as a guide for junior staff in self-improvement.

Serve senior staff as a constant reminder for improvement.

Inventory Categories

The inventory consists of four basic categories: *readability, correctness, appropriateness,* and *thought*. Meaningful subtitles have been listed beneath each broad category. Although the categories are not completely exclusive (some may overlap), the characteristics of each are distinguishable to the extent that one can determine areas of deficiencies and concern.

Readability

Readability, which is nothing more than a clearly understood style of writing, involves judging your audience correctly and writing at a level of their understanding. Not all communication is directed at a general audience and thus, readability styles used for mass media such as journals, newspapers, and even elementary textbooks may not apply to your needs. In addition to judging one's audience, one must assess the complexity and abstractness of the material one is dealing with, and adjust sentence structure accordingly. Whereas a free-flowing flight of style may serve well when the subject is general or concrete, short sentences sticking directly to the subject–verb–object should be used whenever it is important to communicate complex data precisely.

The importance of "paragraph construction" is often overlooked in administrative communication. Long paragraphs permitted in novels and other writings are inappropriate in administrative correspondence. Paragraphs of four or five sentences are generally best. Headings or tables can also be used to create interest.

Topic sentences placed at the beginning of each paragraph make it easier for the reader to grasp the content of the communication quickly. As stated by Fielden (1964), topic sentence use disciplines the writer into including only one main idea in each paragraph.

In letters and reports comprised of thousands of words, it may be necessary to subdivide paragraphs with a topic sentence heading each subdivision serving as a transitional phrase, improving the flow yet maintaining a focus on the important items being discussed in the message.

The use of *jargon*—"shop talk"—can either improve or inhibit readability. The only people who complain about it seriously are those who do not understand it. Jargon is somewhat of a private language effectively employed when all peers relating to the subject understand it. If there is doubt that all persons receiving the communication are familiar with the jargon being used, it is best that it either be translated or replaced by more recognizable language.

Simplicity speaks for itself. Generally speaking, there is no place for the use of unfamiliar words and unusual terms in administrative writing. The use of such unfamiliar terms may be ego gratifying for the writer, and is generally intended to impress either peers or superiors; but such use is often confusing to the reader. Fanciful words should be replaced by simple functional terms that will suffice to explain the message.

Reading direction pertains to the ability of the writer to lead the reader in the right direction through the intricacies of communication. Although generally not pertinent when the message is a short memo reading direction can be vital to the comprehension of complex material. Scientific papers often accomplish this task by briefly abstracting the content of the manuscript and allowing that to precede the document. Often discussion and summary serve to bring into focus a clearer picture of the author's main findings and conclusions. In administrative correspondence, the old rule of "telling your audience what you are about to cover, then cover the subject, and finally tell them what you've told them" still often serves the writer well.

Reading direction is best assured by use of an outline of the content of the correspondence, briefly discussed under the title of "Fundamentals in Writing." For example: The Chancellor requests a statement of needs for faculty and funding for your newly developing Department of Family and Community Medicine. An initial introductory statement could outline the Department's committed responsibilities and might read as follows:

> The Department of Family and Community Medicine has a responsibility for the development of faculty, ancillary support personnel, and facilities for teaching family practice and community medicine in: undergraduate level (pre-clinical and clinical years), graduate level (residents, fellows), continuing medical education for the practicing physician (CME programs), and community and geriatric medicine.

One would then develop a "skeletal frame" (outline) relating to each component that requires definition. As follows:

Department personnel and office facilities. In this instance, the statement could serve as a topic sentence, and within the paragraph there would be a clear definition as to the need for space, secretarial help, equivalent full-time faculty positions, and the approximate cost involved.

Undergraduate education for family practice and community medicine serves as a topic sentence in next paragraph. This could then deal with space for educational purposes, faculty, and ancillary personnel involved and cost.

Continuing medical education for practicing physicians, etc. It should be noted that in each instance, the subdivision relates to the total commitment of the Department and yet clearly defines each component and allows for an easy transition from one item to the next. The statement might end with a short summary as to total faculty positions, total amount of space, and approximate total cost for developing Department activities.

The use of an outline demands that each paragraph flow into the next with a predesigned transitional statement. Also, one should so arrange such elements that the messages of each topic have a close relationship to those that have preceded and those that follow it. Often it helps the reader to understand the main points.

"Focus" is the final aspect of readability. Lack of focus speaks to the confusion caused by superimposing one subject upon another; it describes diffusion of the subject throughout the entire manuscript so that the meaning becomes obscured. Fielden (1964) uses the analogy of an out of focus picture on a TV screen, frequently spoken of as "ghosts." The picture lacks brightness and also clear definition. The writer is challenged to make certain that he has thought through clearly what he means to say and can focus his reader's attention on the salient points.

Correctness

Correctness is the proper use of grammar and punctuation. It must be understood that the ability to write correctly is not synonymous with the ability to write well, and one should not become satisfied with the rather trivial act of mastering punctuation and grammar. Furthermore, the writer must not allow small errors in grammar and punctuation to obscure the true meaning of correctness. It is true that a misplaced comma may occasionally cause confusion but these situations are rare.

The most important aspect of correctness is "coherence"—the proper positioning of elements within a piece of writing so they can be read clearly and sensibly.

Two examples of this concept are as follows:

Incoherent
(1) "I threw the bull over the fence some hay."
(2) "I think it will rain. However, no clouds are showing yet. Therefore, I will take my umbrella."

Coherent
(1) "I threw some hay over the fence to the bull."
(2) "Although no clouds are showing, I think it will rain. Therefore, I will
    take my umbrella."

Once a person has mastered the art of placing related words and
sentences as close as possible to each other, his or her writing will improve
from awkwardness to smoothness. This also requires that paragraphs with
related thoughts be placed next to one another without leapfrogging over
any intervening digressions.

Appropriateness

Appropriateness relates administrative communication to interrelation-
ships of individuals involved in the correspondence process. It involves
those messages going upward or downward in the organization. The
relative position of the writer and the recipient must be recognized and
respected. The difference between a type of communication that a superior
writes to a subordinate, and a type a subordinate writes to the superior
becomes quite obvious.

Upward communication requires "*tact,*" a sensitive perception of what to
say or do to maintain good relationships and to avoid offensiveness. Tact
comes into play when one deals with "style" which will be further
discussed later in this chapter.

A subordinate failing to recognize his role and writing in an argumentative and insulting tone can bring trouble to either himself (or to his boss, if
the directive is sent over the boss's actual or implied signature).

Much time is spent in administration trying to figure out how to tell a
superior he is wrong. When the issue is sensitive, often the best solution is
to discuss the problem on one-to-one level in a comfortable environment
(dinner, lunch, evening meeting) rather than in writing. In preparing a
negative report to a superior it is vital to have details to support your
statements.

Supporting details and opinion require definition according to the writer's
role. In a situation where communication is going upward, it is advisable to
support any statement, especially those of controversy, with considerable
detail. The subordinate soon learns if too much detail is misinterpreted as
inappropriate aggressiveness and will govern himself accordingly by a
more general approach. An indication from above as to the amount of
detail required and desired would be of great value to the writer.

Opinion rendered by a subordinate must be appropriate to the situation
and be carefully thought out to avoid criticism. Occasionally, a superior
wishes a subordinate's opinion. If so, he should so indicate. Failing to do
so, the writer is obligated to indicate clearly where facts cease and opinion
begins, allowing the superior to draw his own conclusions. A better

approach may be to state: "The facts have been presented. I would be willing to render an opinion if desired."

A writer's attitude in an ascending correspondence is very important. Writing with the candor used as if writing to a friend must be guarded against. On the other hand, the writer's choice of words may indicate either too great a desire to impress the boss or an insecurity that imparts a feeling of fearfulness, defenseness, or truculence in the face of authority.

Downward written communication involves persons of higher authority and responsibilities who must relate to subordinates. Unlike in the crafts, trades, or factory industry where assignments relate to specific skills and are straightforward requiring few written messages, the effectiveness of subordinates in upper-level administration, particularly in educational institutions, can be severely limited by an overbearing or insulting message (even without meaning to be). Whereas a subordinate who writes up uses "tact," the superior who writes down must use *"diplomacy."* Although both approaches accomplish somewhat the same objective, tact relates to a sensitive mental perception as to what to do or say to avoid offensiveness. Diplomacy is the art and practice of skillfully negotiating without arousing hostility. Here we have a boss who can *demand*, but *must not*, contrasted to a subordinate who *cannot demand*, but frequently *would like to.*

Furthermore, the superior frequently speaks for the institution, the department, or the company. And any careless message can cause dissension, low productivity, and resignation as well as other human relations problems.

Reliance on power to force compliance rarely achieves positive results for long. More often than not, subordinates resent and resist what they consider arbitrary decisions made by superiors for unknown reasons. It is best if the correspondence explains the reasons for the request and how this benefits the person and the institution involved. The explanations given must be honest, "straight-talk," carefully and tactfully couched in a nonthreatening manner. For example, if a subordinate is requested to take on a new responsibility he or she should be told how the experience will benefit him or her.

Thought

Thought is probably the most basic and certainly the most important category of a "written performance inventory." It is so basic that it frequently gives rise to an angry, defensive retort. "Why, of course I have" when a person is asked, "Have you thought about what you have written?" And yet much disorganized writing results from insufficient thought and failure to identify the purpose and aim of the communication. Most writers think as they write; in fact, many do not recognize a clear thought until it has actually been written down.

Thought is vital in the preparation necessary for establishing your objective for writing, in identifying the reader, and determining the scope of what you would like to say. The real "guts" of administrative writing is intelligent content, and clear thinking sets the stage for the research necessary and the organization of the material to be transmitted. What is the good of an excellent message—readable, correct, and appropriate—if the content is faulty? Much harm can be done despite the fact that one has successfully disguised the communication's superficiality, stupidity, and bias. A superior receiving it may pass it up through the organization with his signature or, worse, may make a disasterous decision based on it.

In considering the thought process that goes into writing, we make the assumption the writer is intellectually competent and capable of the task. If not, a superior must be held responsible for having given his/her assistant a job which is beyond his or her intellectual ability. Thought also involves "*fidelity to the assignment.*" This simply means sticking to the subject and not contaminating the issue by dragging in pet remedies, favorite distortions, or personal axes to grind. Making too much of a routine assignment, usually the characteristic of an eager subordinate, frequently causes lapses in fidelity.

Analysis is probably the most important aspect of the thought process. Often the inexperienced, less intelligent, young administrator will fail because he or she has not analyzed his or her written work. One may not have drawn the obvious conclusion from the data presented; he or she may have drawn conclusions that are not justified by evidence or distorted by bias. A writer who is incapable of making an objective analysis of all sides of the issue will soon lose credibility.

Persuasiveness

To write in a manipulative way to achieve desired results may occasionally be required. Often this approach, if persisted upon, discredits the writer.

It is difficult to describe those qualities that make a communication persuasive: It could be a certain ring of conviction, enthusiasm expressed by the writer, or it could be an understanding of—and appeal to—the reader's desires. It could be from a fine sense of discretion or an action orientation promising results rather than a philosophical approach to the subject. Many things make up a persuasive message.

The propriety of persuasiveness of your communication can be tested by asking yourself whether or not you would care to take action on the basis of what your correspondence presents. If you would be offended or damaged by following your own suggestions, then restate your message. There is no need to concern oneself about routine letters of congratulations or progress reports. But self-testing is imperative for those messages that might cross the line from persuasiveness to bias; these will injure others and so eventually injure you.

Style

Style is integral to effective presentation, interpretation, and response to written messages.

An important part of what you say in a letter or memo is *how you say it*. One could rigidly adhere to all academic rules of writing and fail to convey the message (Hall, 1950). This is true because written communication relates people to one another. It relates to inanimate objects only as they affect persons. Intentions, emphasis, connotation of words, and sentence arrangement are used to communicate not only what you want to say but also how you want the reader to feel before responding.

Styles vary with the occasion. Sometimes it is tactful to be personal, sometimes impersonal. It may feel right to be simple and direct, or wordy and colorful. A passive or forceful approach may suit the occasion at other times. In dealing with style, correct strategy is essential.

Style problems in administrative writing result in volleying drafts of letters and memos back and forth at considerable expense in time, energy and finances. It often gives rise to cries of anguish, "I find it impossible to write letters for my boss's signature. His style is different than mine." "I won't sign a letter if it doesn't sound like me"; "It usually takes my assistant a year to learn my style."

What is the true meaning of style? In an administrative environment various meanings are attached to the word. The definition in Strunk and White's book, *The Elements of Style* (1979),—"The way something is said or done as distinguished from its substance,"—is perhaps how administrators use the word most frequently.

Style is often spoken of as "the way things should be said" or "the tone imparted by the use of words and sentences." In addition to *"denoting,"* words can be used to *"connote,"* which in turn expresses and generates feeling and images.

Whereas literary artists develop and use style for certain expressions, and in so doing, establish valuable identity with certain audiences, administrators write "to get a job done." If a reader dislikes the style of a novelist, he simply does not buy his books. In business, however, an offensive style may prevent a sale, reduce productivity, delay promotion, or give cause for dismissal from one's job. Style can be distinguished, but not divorced from substance. Nor can it be separated from circumstances, likes or dislikes, or the position or power of the reader. Fielden (1982), defines style in business writing as follows:

> Style is that choice of words, sentences and paragraph format which by virtue of being appropriate to the situation and to the power positions of both writer and reader produce the desired reaction and results.

Because of the difficulty in describing what is meant by "style" and how style affects one's administrative writing, a case study protocol described by Fielden (1982) is presented to illustrate various points relating to style. This study concerns *strategy, situations,* and *desired effects* of various styles of administrative writing.

Assume you are an executive in a large computer and software manufacturing company, and you receive the following letter:

Mr. George Apple
Control Data Corporation
Cedar Avenue at 100
Anytown, USA

Dear George:

Over the years of doing business with your company, I have come to respect your professional opinion highly. The advice and service you have provided our University has been very helpful in developing our computer division. I am writing to you now as Chairman of the Finance Committee at our Medical School. We have found it necessary to increase our computer capabilities. I am in the process of establishing an "Ad hoc Committee" of experts to advise us as to what equipment and software will be necessary to meet our needs.

I have suggested that you be included on my Committee as a resource person. I know you will enjoy working with this team of experts in helping us make appropriate decisions for our University. I look forward to your joining us. Let me hear from you soon.

Sincerely,

Mr. Douglas Hanson
Chairman, Finance Committee
University Medical School
Anytown, USA

If you accept the appointment mentioned in this letter, you would have a conflict of interest. As an executive of Control Data, you are certain that your company will submit a proposal to the University for the sale of computer equipment. As President of the University Finance Committee, Mr. Hanson has been a good "software" customer of yours for years. Although he is a well-respected member of your community, you sense that he recognizes the difficult position he has put you in.

Four types of responses can be written to Mr. Hanson's letter, each saying the same thing, but each written in a different style.

Response 1

Mr. Douglas Hanson
Chairman of the Finance Committee
University Medical School
Anytown, USA

Dear Douglas:

You must realize this litigious age often makes it necessary for large companies to take stringent measures not only to avoid conflicts of interest on the part of their employees, but also to preclude even a serious suggestion of conflict. Since my company intends to submit a proposal to your University for the sale of computer equipment, it would not appear appropriate for me to be part of a team responsible for passing judgment on competitor's proposals. Even if I were to excuse myself from consideration of Control Data's proposal, I would be vulnerable to charges that I gave a biased opinion to competitor's offerings.

If there is another way I can serve the Committee and the University that will not raise this conflict of interest issue, you know that I would find it pleasurable to be of service. As always.

Sincerely,

Response 2

Dear Douglas:

Your comments relative to respecting my professional opinion were most appreciated. Furthermore, your invitation to serve on the University's Ad hoc Committee is received with gratitude although with some concern.

The advisory team must be composed of persons free of any allegiance to any vendors submitting proposals. For that reason, it is felt that my services on the Committee could be construed as a conflict of interest.

Perhaps I can be of help in some other way. Again, please be assured that your invitation has been appreciated.

Sincerely,

Response 3

Dear Douglas:

Thank you for suggesting my name as a possible member of your Ad hoc Committee. I wish I could serve, but I cannot.

Control Data would naturally intend to submit a proposal for sale of computer equipment to the University. You can see the position of conflict I would be in if I were on the Advisory Committee.

Just let me know of any other way I can be of service. You know I would be more than willing. Thanks again for the invitation.

Cordially,

Response 4

Dear Doug:

Thanks for the kind words and invitation. Sure wish I could say yes. Can't though.

Control Data intends to submit a sure-fire proposal for computer equipment to the University. Shouldn't be judge and advocate at the same time!

Any other way I can help, Doug, just ask. Thanks again.

Cordially,

Although these four responses might stimulate different reactions in different readers, and although there is enough difference among them to make several relevant points, the message conveyed is the same.

Response 1 seems cold and stilted. The message seems to push the reader away from the writer, and might provoke antagonism. The intellectual quality of word choice seems to parade the writer, while flattering the reader.

Response 2 is very passive and somewhat boring. It presents a cool, impersonal, and somewhat complex attitude of the writer. Despite this, the reaction will probably be neutral (neither strongly positive nor strongly negative). Instead of saying, "I appreciate your comments," it says, "your comments are most appreciated"; instead of "I think my services could be construed as a conflict of interest," it says, "It is felt that my services could be construed, etc., etc."

This is the impersonal passive style of writing characteristic of many individuals with a scientific background. It is harmless, but is certainly not colorful nor is it forceful or interesting.

Response 3 illustrates the style of writing that most high-level executives use. It is like a firm handshake; forceful, warm, simple, and personal. Despite the fact that most administrators like this style, lower-level executives often find themselves afraid to write so forthrightly (and thus find themselves using Responses 1 and 2, believing that style 1 makes them look "smart" to superiors, and style 2, unbossy and fairly impersonal). Those persons who find Response 2 congenial may feel a bit uncomfortable about the appropriateness of Response 3. One gets the impression that more readers in *high positions* would like Response 3 than would readers who are in *lower positions*.

Response 4 is annoyingly self-confident and breezy, going far beyond being forceful. Because it is so conversational, it presents an intense personal and warm feeling that many business people would find offensive. This is true even with very close acquaintances such as Mr. Doug Hanson. It has the tone of an advertiser's chant.

Strategy and Style

What difference does it make which style I use? A style used in one situation may be inappropriate in another. Circumstances not only alter situations but also alter *you*. Thus, at times, it may be wise to be forceful, and at other times being forceful may be self-destructive. It is occasionally appropriate to be colorful, and at other times this approach is ludicrous. To be personal or impersonal must be carefully weighed, depending on the situation. Keep in mind that individuals who write effectively have no single style for all circumstances and readers, and instead they select the style that fits a particular reader and situation.

In administration people often face one or more of the following writing situations: *Positive situations*—saying yes or conveying good news. *Situations where some action is asked of the reader*—giving orders or persuading someone to do as requested. *Information—conveying situations*—for example, describing a course curriculum. *Negative situations*—saying no or relaying bad news. The choice of style in each situation may be of *strategic* importance.

In a *"positive situation,"* because readers are often so pleased to hear pleasant news, style is sometimes ignored. Yet such news communicated by the writer in a cold, impersonal, roundabout, begrudging manner may upset the reader.

Action requests usually involve negotiating. If the writer holds power, he/she can use a more forceful, commanding style. However, this must be done with diplomacy. A writer, usually a subordinate with no power over the reader, must use extreme tact. If actions are asked for, the reader must be persuaded and not ordered. A forceful style here would be unsuitable.

Information—conveying situations usually are not emotionally charged. Thus, getting the message across in a straightforward manner is usually best.

Negative situations require diplomacy at its best. Correct style here depends on the relationship of the person being told "no" to that person saying "no." Relating to the example presented if you were Mr. Apple you would be forced to deny the request of a very good customer. Having sensed that Mr. Hanson has placed you in a potential conflict of interest, your "no" answer would require a tactful style.

This brings up the issue of *"situations form the basis of style selection,"* again, taking from Fielden (1982), in the previously presented case study. "Do we want to be personal and warm? Usually yes, but in this situation? Do we want to communicate clearly, directly, and forcefully? Usually yes, but here? Do we want to appear as if we're brushing aside the conflict, as the third response does? Or do we want to approach that issue longwindedly, as the first response, or passively as in the second? What is the strategically appropriate style?" It is in situations such as these that accurately judging the appropriate response separates the successful from the unsuccessful executive communicators.

With strategy in mind, we note that the first response transforms the personal nature of the communication into a formal statement. The message has an abstract, textbook like sound that downplays the tone of personal rejection. This is done by use of legalistic phrases and Latin vocabulary. It successfully draws the writer back from being close to the reader.

In reviewing Response 2, the lack of personal warmth appears to be correct for the situation. By using the passive constantly, the writer draws back and avoids the need to say, "I must say no." The word construed reinforces the passive. Although this letter seems dull and lacking personal warmth, for the situation that involves a potentially unethical action, despite our likes and dislikes, it is an appropriate response.

The third and fourth responses strategically do not fit the situation. The direct nature of the responses, although colorful, point out the obvious conflict and may prove offensive in such a sensitive situation.

The *wanted effect* in style may be difficult to accomplish. Style varies with situations and one must learn to write in several styles. A warm, personal, and colorful style should be used in a letter to be read before a group honoring a retiring friend. A long analytical report may require a passive, impersonal style. Yet, a very forceful style is called for in a persuasive memo asking for recommendations.

Common Styles

From Fielden (1982), six of the most common styles used in administrative writings will be presented. These styles are forceful, passive, personal, impersonal, colorful, and less colorful.

Forceful Style

A forceful style is usually appropriate only in a downward communication where the writer has power, such as in action requests, in the form of orders or when one is saying "no" firmly, but politely to a subordinate.

> One should use the active voice. Your statements are designed to do something to people and objects, and not the reverse. Often this takes the form of giving orders; 'correct this mistake immediately' (the subject understood is you) instead of 'a correction should be made...' (which leaves the reader wondering made by whom).
> One should be honest, and forthright: 'I have decided to dismiss you from your job' instead of, 'Unfortunately, it has been recommended that you be discharged from your present position.'
> As often as possible, your sentences should be written in a simple subject, verb object order. Do not weaken them by putting inappropriate modifying

phrases before the subject. 'I have decided to lend you the necessary money for your project' instead of 'after much consultation, deliberation, and weighing the positives and negatives, I have decided to lend you the necessary finances for your project.'

A forceful style demands confidence and security in the tone you adapt. Do not use modifiers such as 'possibly,' 'maybe,' 'perhaps,' 'it could be concluded that,' 'some might conclude that.'

Passive Style

A passive style is generally used in a negative situation or in situations where the writer is in a lower position and is communicating up to the reader.

It is imperative never to give an order using the passive style.

Avoid the imperative. Direct statements such as: 'Present your report more clearly at our next meeting,' 'time is valuable, get right to the point' should be avoided. Instead, 'it is necessary to devise a more effective and time-conserving method of presenting your report before our next meeting.'

The use of long sentences and complex paragraphs will slow down the reader's comprehension of sensitive or negative information.

The use of passive voice tends to subordinate the subject. This is especially effective if one is in a low power position and is required to convey negative information to the reader who is in a higher position (superior, customer, very important persons). Instead of saying 'You are wasting valuable resources,' Say, 'valuable resources are being wasted.' It is best to say, 'Several objections might be raised by those hostile to your plans' instead of 'I have several objections to your plans.' By so doing, you avoid taking responsibility for negative statements by attributing them to a faceless, impersonal 'other.'

Personal Style

This style is usually appropriate in good news and persuasive "action— request situations."

In this situation, one would use the active voice which puts one as the writer in front of the sentence: 'I appreciated your comments' instead of 'your comments were very much appreciated by me.' First names should be used when appropriate, instead of referring to individuals by title: "John Jones attended the meeting" instead of 'Mobil's Director attended the meeting.'

Use of personal pronouns, especially 'you' and 'I' when you are saying positive things. 'I so much appreciate the work you've done' as opposed to 'The work you've done is appreciated.'

A personal touch can be added by using contractions (can't, won't, shouldn't).

The use of short sentences that mimic ordinary conversation is appropriate. 'I discussed your idea with Frank, he's all for it!' as opposed to, 'This is to inform you that your idea was taken up at Thursday's meeting and that it was regarded with favor.'

An interjection of a positive personal thought such as: 'How are Mary and the kids?' will make the reader know that this letter is really directed at him/her, and is not a form letter reproduced from a word processing instrument.

Impersonal Style

The impersonal style is often used to convey negative information and for technical and scientific writings. In these situations, one rarely uses the person's name, but refers to individuals by their title or job description: "our vice president of finances" or "the finance department," not "Mrs. Smith."

Personal pronouns, especially 'you and I' should be avoided. 'We wonder if the idea will work' rather than 'I don't think the idea will work.' A convenient method of making yourself disappear when desired is to use the passive voice. 'A mistake in the numbers has been made' instead of 'I think you've made a mistake in the numbers you've recorded.' In these situations, your sentences may be complex and your paragraphs as long as necessary. Avoid the short, brisk, direct, simple style of conversation.

Colorful Style

In good news situations, a lively colorful style is most desirable. This style is frequently found in highly persuasive writings of sales letters and advertisements.

Adjectives and adverbs are used profusely. Instead of, "This engineer will save the organization money," one might write, "This highly motivated, intelligent engineer will surely save our hard-earned, increasingly scarce company finances."

Less Colorful Style

A less colorful style is more appropriate for ordinary business writing, and also for much administrative correspondence in educational institutions. By minimizing the use of adjectives, adverbs, and figures of speech, one can become unemotionally involved with the ordinary written communicating tasks of the day.

This is a blending of the passive and impersonal style. Wit, liveliness, and vigor are generally inappropriate in the use of this style.

Style Guidelines

The six styles depicted by Fielden are not mutually exclusive. There is overlap among them frequently. However, there are sufficient distinct features of each style that distinguishes one from the other and permits one to relate various styles to situations and circumstances. It must be remembered as stated by Fielden (1982), that "(1) each style has an impact on the reader, (2) style communicates to readers almost as much as the content of the message, (3) style cannot be isolated from the situation, (4) generalizing about which style is the best in all situations is impossible, (5) style must be altered to suit the circumstances, (6) style must be discussed sensibly in the work situation."

Control of one's style and the engineering of the tone of the written communication can make one's written correspondence more effective. Alvarez (1980) provides a summary of guidelines which, if followed, would accomplish much in the improvement of style in administrative communication. These are listed as follows:

> Be selective; focus on the essential information, the significant detail.
> Develop a lean, direct style; avoid inflated language and rambling sentences.
> Write in the present tense whenever possible for simplicity and immediacy.
> Use examples and comparisons to clarify descriptions and explanations.
> Repeat words or phrases for clarity or emphasis, or to erase transitions; but avoid needless repetition.
> Delete needless words and phrases, but avoid shortcuts that sacrifice meaning.
> Choose clarity over style if they conflict.

Written Communication Considered as a Mechanical Skill

A mechanical skill is usually viewed as a performance involving a series of set repeated steps and often these steps can be listed or diagrammed in ways easy for others to understand (Sale, 1970). Although mechanical skills in writing include all aspects involved in the use of the written word, the following material will summarize only the salient points in the use of words, sentences, paragraphs, punctuation, and grammar in administrative writing. A brief review of the principles of administrative writing according to Alvarez (1980) would state "that the basic function of administrative writing is to inform; the form and tone will depend on its purpose and audience; accuracy, clarity, coherence and conciseness are essential qualities."

Words used in administrative correspondence must be selected for clarity and power. Each word used must be considered in relation to its possible impact on the reader. Avoid misuse of adjectives and adverbs and use one only if it adds precision or dimension to the word it modifies. Short words are preferable to long ones. Avoid the use of clichés, euphemisms, and jargon. The use of a dictionary ensures accuracy; a thesaurus increases vocabulary.

The variable types of sentences and their appropriate use within written communication comes with experience. What is important, however, is that the sentence structure does not distort or destroy the meaning of your intended message. For various forms of communication, special sentence structures are frequently required. For a detailed description of the appropriate use of sentences, see *The Elements of Technical Writing* by Joseph Alvarez (1980).

Punctuation occupies a position of lesser prominence in the discussion of the appropriate methods and skills of administrative correspondence. The use of punctuation is important, but is in a constant state of change. Modern punctuation has become simpler, and one tends to punctuate less and less, and only when necessary. The written language—what it does and how well it does it—counts more on form and tone than on punctuation. The purpose of punctuation is first to clarify and second to create rhythm. Thus, a rudimentary knowledge of punctuation from any elementary grammar text would suffice for the writer's purposes.

Communication Instruments

The specific format selected for administrative writing is determined by the purpose of the writer and the writer's audience. The traditional written structure usually includes (1) an introduction, (2) body, and (3) a conclusion. The introduction orients the reader, it includes necessary background information, and describes the intent and the scope of the written piece. The body contains *the what, how*, and *why* of the subject. The conclusion pulls everything said into focus and ties it all together. In the conclusion the writer summarizes and if necessary evaluates, discusses, and recommends.

As stated by Alvarez (1980), "there are no universal rules of format, but one basic precaution is worth remembering: format should serve the writer, not vice-versa."

The written instruments of communication can take several forms: reports, directions, procedural instructions, resumes, letters of inquiry, etc. Correspondence can be of a formal form institutional letter, a memo, or a personal letter. Other communication writings will relate to the objective to be accomplished by the communication sent and the communicator's intent.

Physical appearance of the particular piece of writing such as; "full blocked letter style, semi-blocked or indented style" (Fig. 6-1), whether or not it contains a company's letterhead is not important. But neatness and organization of the material are important. The type style used should be simple and readable. Memoranda forms are frequently provided by the institution. One may wish to use a handy reference dealing with the mechanical details of writing, such as Gavin and Sabin's (1970) *Reference Manual for Stenographers and Typists*.

Administrative letters and memos have always been an extremely formal method of communication. Today, however, written correspond-

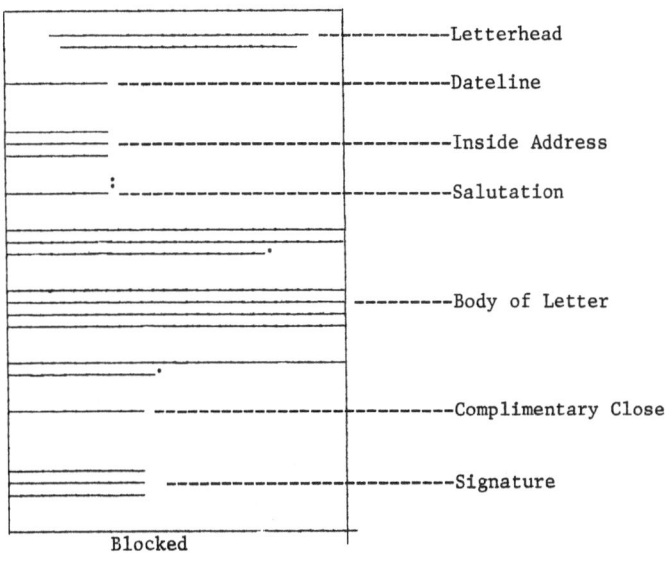

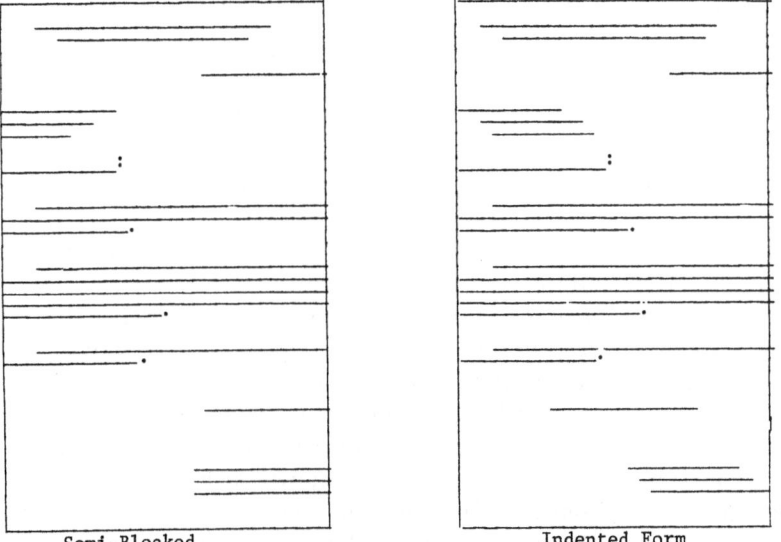

Figure 6-1. Letter formats.

ence has become more conversational and informal. Contracts or other legal documents written in letter form are still very rigid and impersonal. Most administrative letters—whether they concern business, technical writings or reports—serve to inform. But many persuade and some instruct. Still others combine these functions. Regardless of the instrument used and for what purpose there are no short cuts to achieving clarity in letter and memorandum writing. This objective can be accomplished only by the application of the fundamentals of writing previously described.

Personal Correspondence
(Administrative and/or Business Letters)

There are almost as many "types" of letters as there are reasons for writing them. Several will be listed as model examples.

Regardless of the format used, a business letter consists of six parts. They are (1) heading, (2) inside address, (3) salutation, (4) body of the letter, (5) closing, which consists of the complimentary close and the signature (handwritten then typed), and (6) any added notations.

(1) The heading of the letter gives the full address of the writer and the date of the letter.
(2) The inside address gives the name and full address of the addressee.
(3) The salutation greets the addressee appropriately.

The salutation should be consistent with the tone of the letter, the first line of the inside and the complimentary close.

When the surname of the addressee is known, it is used in the salutation of the business letter as in the following examples: Dear Dr. Davis:, Dear Mrs. Greer:, Dear Mayor Smith:, Dear Ms. Joseph.

If there is doubt as to what preference a woman would choose to be addressed, use Ms., which is always appropriate. In letters to organizations or persons whose name and sex are unknown such salutations as the following are customary: Dear Sir or Madam:, Dear Subscription Manager:, Dear Registrar. If you do not know the name of the addressee but you do know the sex, use either Dear Sir or Dear Madam. The appropriate form of salutation and address in letters to government officials, legislative persons, military personnel varies according to the office or persons involved. Often such information is available in the dictionaries cited in the bibliography.

(4) The body of the letter should follow the principles of good writing as previously described.
(5) The closing ends the letter. The complimentary close can be extremely formal or less formal. Commonly in formal situations, one uses "very

truly yours," "yours truly," or "sincerely yours." In instances less formal use "sincerely" or "cordially." It is important in all business correspondence that the name and title of the sender be typed below the signature.

(6) Notations supply additional information, such as whether anything is enclosed with the letter, to whom copies of the letters have been sent (cc: AAW, PTN) and the initials of the sender and the typist (DM/CLL) (see Table 6-2).

Various types of personal letters are required for effective administrative communication. Some of the most common forms will be described.

Letters to Legislators and/or Public Officials

Administrators in all fields, especially medical education, must often write to their state or federal legislators and other public officials. Some cardinal rules will help assure a favorable reception to your letter:

Respect the office. It is important to use an appropriate title, address, and salutation such as:

The Honorable Robert Dole
United States Senate
2213 Dirksen Senate Office Building
Washington, D.C.

Dear Senator Dole:

Respect the reader's time. Public officials, especially Congressmen, receive hundreds of letters from their constituents. It is impossible for them to read all such correspondence. This is frequently done by other people who very soon recognize appropriate requests. Do not write unless your reason is meaningful. Problems that are persistent and progressive must be addressed, but writing often regarding trivial concerns reduces the impact of a worthwhile request.

Be specific as to why you are writing. Unless officials and legislators are personal friends a strict adherence to the formal protocol previously described will serve you best. Your introduction should state simply why you are writing, i.e., "I am writing concerning the reduced appropriations for graduate medical education for family practice residencies."

Clearly state your cause. The body of your letter should clearly and briefly state your message. Present a short historical perspective, your concern, and what you would have the official do.

Leave a legacy of good will. It is in this portion of the letter that you can reinforce some common bonds. This could be of a personal or semi-personal nature and end with a favorable complimentary close, i.e., "It was

Table 6-2. Indented Format of Model Business Letter

STATE	MEDICAL	COLLEGE

1984 Beard Avenue   Anytown, USA 92486

                                                          State Medical College
                                                          1984 Beard Avenue
(Doublespace twice)   Anytown, USA 92486
March 6, 1983 ◄————————— Date with Letterhead or—►March 6, 1983
(Doublespace)   Stationery
John Harris, M.D.
Community Health Center   ⎤—Inside Address
5608 Weston Avenue
Anytown, USA 56093   ⎦
(Doublespace)
Dear Dr. Harris: Salutation   P
(Doublespace)   A
   [Introductory paragraph. It should establish contact with the reader.]   I   R
Such as: We have just completed reviewing the outline sent to us for   N   A
involving our students in a community health educational program in   T   G
your center. We are very pleased with its content.   R   R
(Doublespace)   O   A
   [The body of the letter should consist of paragraphs with single spacing   P
within and double spacing between them.] Such as: I am impressed with   H
the total format which includes didactic lectures and seminars of cognitive
material relating to epidemiology, population disease and common health
responsibilities.   B
(Doublespace)   O
   I was particularly impressed with the addition of educational material   D
you are offering concerning care of the elderly.   Y
(Doublespace)
   Your attention to "wellness" and "health maintenance" is indeed a
desired addition to our curriculum. Etc., etc.
(Doublespace)   C   P
   [The concluding paragraph should summarize, direct, propose, sug-   O   A
gest, and/or leave a legacy of goodwill with the reader if possible.] Such N   R
as: The material you forwarded to us demonstrated much research and   C   A
work on the part of your staff. We plan to work your suggestions into our   L   G
undergraduate curriculum. I'll be contacting you shortly in this matter.   U   R
We look forward to working with you.   D   A
      (Doublespace)   I   P
                                                                           N   H
                                                                           G

                              Sincerely,   Complimentary close   C
                                                                                                    L
                                                                                                    O
                              Signature   S
(Doublespace twice)   D.J. James, M.D.   Typed name   I
                      Chairman, Department of   Title   N
                      Family Medicine   G
(Doublespace)
DM/ewl   Notation

my pleasure to visit with your friend, John Smith, the other day; he asked me to send his greetings. With best personal regards."

In Appreciation of (Thank you Letter)

Thank you letters serve very useful purposes in business and administration. Such a letter may be handwritten to add a personal touch. However, use of an informal, indented style on official stationery will add the prestige of your institutional office and yet fulfill the requirement for a more personal touch. Such letters should be brief, avoiding adherence to a strict protocol, and should carry a very forthright message. An example:

Richard Walsh, M.D., Dean
604 Drew Drive
Wichita, Kansas 21304

Dear Dean Walsh:

Thank you very much for recommending me to Alpha Omega Alpha Honor Society. I appreciate your support and encouragement over the last four years.

Sincerely,

Jim Freemont

Letter of Transmittal

A letter of transmittal—generally a cover letter accompanying an article or report—could be a formal letter or may take the form of an informal memorandum. It should include (1) the subject of the report, (2) authorizations for the report, (3) an offer to answer any questions the recipient may have, and (4) an acknowledgment of any assistance received in the preparation of the report. It may also include additional information, depending on the specific circumstances.

Claim and Adjustment Letter

One of the most common business letters is one of claim and adjustment. It must include, above all else, your specific claim and what you request be done in the disposition of the matter.

Your claim should describe exactly what is wrong. The more specific the description, the easier and the quicker it will be corrected. Your claim may involve a transport company that has lost a piece of equipment or it may involve the loss of a suitcase in an airline, or a piece of appliance that has been faulty. In each instance specific information as to the type of equipment, the model, the serial numbers and the brand name and style must be included.

The company involved in this transaction will often be more than happy to satisfy your demands. To be specific and reasonable in your request is of utmost importance.

Order Letter

The success of an order letter depends on supplying precise information: a description of the product with specific model or stock number, page of the catalog, quantity of each item, price, and indication of destination. Clearly identify where the order is to be shipped and any special considerations such as whether the order must be shipped on a specific date or in a particular way (freight, air, parcel post). Be sure to include the payment or tell how the merchandise is to be paid for.

Letter of Inquiry

One or more of the common uses for administrative writing is to obtain information. The letter of inquiry usually poses an imposition on the individual that you are requesting this information from thus deserves special attention. It can be a simple note requesting a free brochure or as complex as "A Protocol for Self-evaluation of Faculty."

The more complicated the letter the more carefully it must be constructed. Few things are more frustrating than failing to receive the answer to the question you thought you asked, but did not. Your second letter might not get a prompt response or any response at all.

Since the letter of inquiry asks for a response by the reader, you must state what you want, who needs it, why it is needed, and how it is to be used; specific questions must be easy to answer. And finally, an expression of your appreciation is imperative. If possible indicate to the recipient how he will either benefit by supplying this information or offer a favor in return. A stamped self-addressed envelope encourages a prompt response.

Letter of Technical Information

This type of letter differs from others in that it is, in effect, a short technical report. It may take the form of a memorandum for use within the department or it may be a letter or a report to another institution. Since this letter or memo in many instances deals with specific detailed information, it is most helpful to the reader if you clearly state the purpose. A clear definition on every point must be made. The writer must follow the appropriate steps in the writing process that relate to introduction, body, and conclusion.

Instruments for Faculty and/or Personnel Recruitment

Application Letters

The letter of application, one of the most common forms of administrative correspondence, is essentially a sales letter (Hall, 1950). One is trying to sell his or her services with competition from other applicants. Therefore the letter of application must do three things: (1) catch the reader's attention in a favorable way, (2) create a desire for your services, (3) ask for an interview.

This is one of the most difficult letters to write. It must both inform and persuade. The writer must steer a narrow course between sounding boastful and seeming ordinary. Since this letter may be one of the most important bits of written communication that you have ever written, specific guidelines would apply here: (1) establish contact with the reader, (2) be specific and direct, yet thorough and concise; (3) use personal pronouns; (4) keep paragraphs short; (5) cite reasons and evidence why you qualify for the job; (6) emphasize the benefits to the employer for hiring you; and (7) do not promise more than you can deliver (Alvarez, 1980).

Before you write, however, you must ask yourself who you are and what you want. There must be a recognition on the part of the writer as to his or her special qualities, strengths, and limitations. If the job calls for a leader or a follower, an outgoing or an introverted person, do you fit into those categories? What are your personal goals: wealth, excitement, prestige, glamour, freedom, challenging work, security, fame, or power? The message as to why you want the job must be clearly conveyed in a manner that not only informs but also persuades. All personal information (education, work history, etc.) can be conveniently documented on a separate data sheet as a curriculum vitae or a résumé (to be discussed later).

In your letter, it is important to:

(1) State that you are applying for a specific job, not just any job, and indicate where you learned about the position;
(2) Give specific information showing that you are qualified for the specific job;
(3) Stress your qualifications and refer the reader to your resume for less important details;
(4) Ask for an interview. Make it as convenient as possible for your prospective employer. State when and where you can be reached and when you will be available for the interview. Remember, employers hire for their own reasons, not for the applicant's. So keep the reader's, the prospective employer's, point of view in mind.

Pay careful attention to such details as:

Address the letter to a person rather than a department, if possible. The correct name and title can be obtained by telephoning local representatives, various institutions or personnel departments.

Make certain that your letter and résumé are accurate as to facts, spelling, and grammar.

Neatness is of utmost importance. Your typewriter should be clean and no smudges should occur on your written material. If you do not type well have someone who does type well do the letter for you.

Use good quality paper. It will prove to be an excellent investment.

Résumé Formulation

A "résumé," "vitae," or the personal "data sheet" is a historical record of your professional activities. In effect, a résumé is a catalog of what you have to offer a prospective employer. It is the basis for their decision to invite you for a personal interview. It should in an orderly, readable, and easy to understand fashion tell them who you are, what you know, what you can do, what you have done, and what your job objectives are (Hall, 1950).

The résumé is an important document from the employer's standpoint also. It serves as a focus for the interview, aids in evaluating the interview after the applicant's departure, and serves as an organized reminder of what was discussed during the interview.

Three steps are involved in preparing and using a résumé effectively. First is to analyze yourself and your background; the second is to organize and prepare the resume; third is to identify those to whom you will submit the instrument.

In analyzing yourself and background, you must research thoroughly your experience, education and training, and personal traits.

There is always a question as to how detailed a résumé should be. In my experience, having interviewed scores of prospective candidates for many administrative and teaching positions, the résumé needs to be all-inclusive. I believe that an individual should compile a résumé early in his or her professional lifetime, then modify it with additions and subtractions as the position applied for dictates. Taken from Brusaw et al. (1976), the following outlines serve as an excellent guide in the development of a resume.

Experience—List and describe all past employment including full-time and part-time jobs and free-lance work according to the following questions.
(1) What was the job title?

(2) What did you do (in reasonable detail)?

(3) What experience did you gain that you can apply to other jobs?

(4) Why were you hired for the job?

(5) What special skills did you develop on the job?

(6) When did you start and when did you leave the job?

(7) Why did you leave the job?

(8) Would your former employer give you a reference?

(9) What special traits were required of you on the job (initiative, leadership, ability to work with details, ability to work with people, imagination, ability to organize, etc.)?

Education—for both the recent graduate with little work experience and the person with an extensive job background, education, and training constitute a very important part of a resume. The following information about your education should be listed in detail.

(1) Schools attended with inclusive dates.

(2) Degrees and the dates they were awarded.

(3) Major and minor subjects.

(4) Courses taken or skills acquired that might be especially pertinent to the job now being applied for.

(5) Cumulative scholastic average and any academic honors.

(6) Extracurricular activities.

(7) Scholarships and awards.

(8) Special training (academic or industrial).

Personal characteristics—There are several reasons for listing your personal characteristics. In doing so you will be evaluating yourself as to your strengths and weaknesses, and your suitability for the job you seek. It aids in assessing the job in relation to your future professional growth. The points to consider are:

(1) Age and marital status, children if any.

(2) Height, weight, health and physical limitations.

(3) Communication skills.

(4) Social attitudes (aggressive, cooperative, cheerful, tactful, moody, and courteous).

(5) Career objectives and plans for the future.

Organizing and writing a resume should be done in relation to the job one is seeking. After evaluating all items, you will soon reject some of them, finally selecting those that you will include in the final resume. Base your decision as to what is rejected and what is kept by asking the following questions:

(1) Precisely what job are you seeking?

(2) Who is the prospective employer?

(3) What information is most pertinent to the job and that employer?

(4) What details should be included and in what order?

(5) How can you present your qualifications most effectively to get an interview?

There are many guidelines that can be used in organizing the information that you wish to submit. The most common is the listing of the jobs held starting with the most recent and going back to the first. It is important that the succession of jobs and promotions, including titles and responsibilities, be clearly delineated. The second most common way to organize a resume is by function. This is accomplished by starting with the function most closely related to the job being applied for, followed by the next most relevant and so on. Again in this instance, it is important to describe each function using specific illustrations of your experience. Examples of résumés of various types can be found in Brusaw et al.'s (1976) *Handbook of Technical Writing.*

Outline of Recruitment Interview

The process of interviewing a candidate becomes a muddle unless an individual has some basic outline that allows for categorizing specific information that one hopes to derive from the interview process. Table 6-3 is an example of an outline which will, within broad categories, remind the interviewer of the subjects that must be covered in the interview process. The completed interview outline combined with a previous résumé will provide the prospective employer with desired detailed information concerning the candidate.

Table 6-3.   Guide for Interviewing Potential Faculty for the Department of Family Medicine

---

Credentials related to stated job description

Personality

Behavioral adaptive potential: Will the candidate be able to satisfactorily integrate, relate and function within the faculty structure?

Growth potential within the department and university structure

---

Letters of Reference

Using the standard business letter format, a letter of reference should include portions of all that is contained in a résumé. It is important to discuss four broad categories: the applicant's credentials in relation to the job description; personality; behavioral adaptive ability to area and individuals; and growth potential. A letter of reference, if it is to be fair to the previous employee and the prospective employer, must be forthright, concise, and clear.

Job Description Format

A job description format will vary depending on the position being offered. In a medical teaching institution, it is necessary that one specify the various categories of activities that the prospective employee is expected to be involved in. The percentage of time spent in each activity is important in allowing the prospective employee to judge whether or not he or she is qualified for (or interested in) the position. Table 6-4 is a model job description.

Letter of Acceptance

When one has received an offer of a job, it is important that a letter of acceptance be submitted immediately. The format for such a letter should be simple, stating that it is with pleasure that you are accepting the job that has been offered. One must guard against being too exuberant or overly gracious in accepting the offer. It is important that you identify the job you are accepting and state the salary and the conditions of the acceptance so there is no confusion on these points. This then becomes a document that can be placed in a personnel file for future reference. If necessary, a second paragraph might go into the details of moving and reporting for the position accepted. The letter should be completed with a statement of "legacy of pleasure" in looking forward to working for your new employer. It is important to use a style that will maintain a degree of formality and yet demonstrate personal warmth.

Letter of Refusal

A letter of refusal must include an introductory statement specifically stating that you have refused the position, such as: "I am sorry I cannot accept your offer as a junior faculty person for undergraduate education in family medicine." This then sets the stage for the second paragraph in which you may want to make a few statements as to the reasons why you cannot accept the position. Regardless of the reasons why you are not accepting the position and the personal attitudes involved in your making that decision it is appropriate that a formal, warm, and cordial attitude be

Table 6-4. Job Description

Position
Director of Family Practice Residency Program at St. Joseph Medical Center
Qualifications
M.D. degree, Board Certified or Board Qualified, Diplomat status
Preferred qualifications
Five (5) years experience as faculty person active in a Family Practice Residency
Responsibilities or duties
The Program Director has administrative, educational, service, and research responsibilities.
Administrative (40%):
  (1) Responsible for the operation of the Family Practice Residency Program including the Family Practice Center.
  (2) Report monthly at Family and Community Medicine Departmental meeting.
Educational (30%):
  (1) Responsible for coordinating, implementing, and updating the core curriculum of the residents educational experiences within the program in keeping with requirements of ACGME.
  (2) Share responsibilities with other full-time and part-time faculty.
    (a) Make morning and evening rounds as required with residents.
    (b) Make teaching rounds, not less than every second day.
    (c) Coordinate resident activities in relation to the team approach to medicine.
    (d) Regulate and coordinate outpatient activities such as emergency room, clinic experiences in doctor's office and similar educational site.
    (e) Arrange for one out-of-residency postgraduate study experience of one or two months for each resident during his second and third years.
    (f) Responsible for the needs of the resident in relation to family and community.
    (g) Develop system to review daily the clinical experience on every patient seen by PL-1, every second patient seen by PL-2 and randomly review activities of PL-3.
Service (20%):
  (1) Responsible for the health care needs of all patients who are registered at the Family Practice Center.
  (2) Establish a private practice and see patients at least three half-days per week.
  (3) Together with other full-time faculty participate in evening and week-end coverage of the private practice.
Research (10%):
  Establish the means by which research and analysis within available research time can be performed by members of the full-time and part-time faculty as well as the household staff. Serve as a leader in research projects.

---

conveyed. There is nothing to be gained by being abrupt or rude in your *not* accepting a position. It is important to remember that letters are documents that frequently are filed for future reference. The complimentary close should again leave a "legacy of pleasure" with your reader.

Summary: Types of Letters

The following guide is a summary of what is to be included in various types of letters using the basic format and fundamentals previously described.

Simple Request:
(1) A courteously stated explanation for writing.
(2) The request itself, along with any further explanation that may be needed by the reader.
(3) A courteous ending, indicating urgency if necessary.

Multiple-Question Inquiry
(1) A courteously stated explanation for writing.
(2) The request for information, made in a generalized statement that points to:
(3) A list of clear, specific questions, numbered in sequence and set off from the rest of the letter.
(4) An invitation to send any additional information that may be helpful.
(5) A courteous ending, indicating urgency if necessary.

Yes and No Replies
(1) A courteous acknowledgment of the request.
(2) A complete explanation presented before the refusal.
    (But, be careful here. There are times when a complete explanation is not advisable. If you are in doubt, check with someone who knows more.)
(3) An indication of an effort to demonstrate empathy, if possible.
(4) A courteous ending, perhaps with a little statesmanship and, if necessary, a statement of regret.

Orders
(1) How many?
(2) What unit?
(3) What product name?
(4) What size?
(5) What price?
(6) Means of transportation
(7) Date shipment desired

Claims and Complaints
(1) A courteously stated listing of the most significant details.

(2) A presentation of all facts pointing to the claim itself.
(3) A clear-cut statement of the adjustment desired.
(4) A reasonable argument substantiating the request for adjustment and motivating the reader to comply.
(5) A courteous ending, perhaps with the writer's offer to do something to obtain prompt adjustment. (BUT, no one likes to be threatened.)
Responding to Claims and Complaints
(1) Be careful, check, if necessary, with superiors and lawyers.
(2) Include an explanation.
(3) Include the company's adjustment, if any.
(4) Be courteous and empathic; the customer is already angry.

Memoranda

The most common type of administrative business and industrial communication is the memorandum or "memo." The appropriate use of memos for internal communication saves considerable time and effort on the part of administrative personnel. The memo is immediate, concise, and almost telegraphic. It may vary from two lines to two pages, but rarely more. Whereas letters are used to correspond outside of an institution, memos are used within a department, institution, or company. Often standard memo forms are printed with specific headings which outline what is to be included. As stated by Alvarez (1980): "A memo can be the most formal of formats." However, it can also have an informal connotation depending on the style with which it is written and whether or not it is an "up" or "down" communication.

Because of the nature of the memo it need not establish direct contact with the reader. The contact is already made by the nature of the instrument used to communicate. A common printed format is as follows:

```
DATE:     January 6, 1983
TO:       Matt Johnson
FROM:     Jack Smith
SUBJECT:  Evaluation Instrument for Undergraduate Education

cc: Jim O'Donnell
    Tom Frasier
```

A memo should be used when the subject is minor or of passing importance, or is a single aspect of a larger project. Without the use of salutation, state the message of the memo, develop it as concisely and clearly as possible, and add any recommendations or conclusions. There is no need for a complimentary close or signature.

Conclusion

The ability to effectively communicate by written correspondence in administration requires transmitting a message accurately, clearly, and appropriately. This demands that the writer understand the basic fundamentals of good writing as well as style, strategies, situations, and mechanics used in the writing process. Using the concepts and models described in the preceding chapter will help an administrator communicate more effectively using written correspondence.

Faculty Development Activities

(1) If you were the recipient of a letter of reference, list the major items you would like to read in the letter. Compare your lists of the letter for a faculty applicant versus a residency applicant.
(2) Outline your approach to writing negative letters of references. Discuss your approach with other faculty members. Why is it so difficult or undesirable to write such letters?
(3) Review your daily administrative correspondence patterns. What types of communication (i.e., memos, letters of reference, administrative letters) do you write most frequently?
   (a) Randomly select two items of each type and analyze using the "Written Performance Inventory."
   (b) Using the same items, review your predominant style(s) (forceful, passive, personal, impersonal, colorful, less colorful).
(4) Select several pieces of administrative correspondence you have received. Decipher the predominant style(s) which the author used. Decide how the style affected your reaction to the contents of the correspondence.
(5) During the coming week, plan your strategy for the content and style of your administrative correspondence. Prior to writing, outline your content and decide on desired style(s). Analyze the finished written correspondence using the "Written Performance Inventory."

References

Alvarez JA. The elements of technical writing. New York: Harcourt, Brace, Jovanovich, 1980.

The American heritage dictionary of the English language. Boston: American Heritage and Houghton Mifflin, 1969.

Brusaw CT, Alred GJ, Aliu WE. Handbook of technical writing. New York: St. Martin's Press, 1976.

The Chicago manual of style. Chicago: University of Chicago Press, 1982.

Fielden JS. What do you mean you don't like my style? Harvard Business Review, May–June 1982:128–38.

Fielden JS. What do you mean I can't write? Harvard Business Review, May–June 1964:144–56.

Gavin RE, Sabin WA. Reference manual for stenographers and typists. New York: McGraw–Hill Book Company, 1970.

Hall, M. Getting your ideas across through writing. Washington, D.C.: U.S. Department of Health, Education and Welfare, 1950.

Hodges JC, Whitten MD. Harbrace college handbook, 9th ed. New York: Harcourt, Brace, Jovanovich, 1982:517–27.

Moore WE. The conduct of the corporation. New York: Random House, 1962:72–3.

Randle CW. How to identify promotable executives. Harvard Business Review, May–June 1956:122.

Sale R. On writing. New York: Random House, 1970.

Strunk W Jr, White B. The elements of style. New York: Macmillan, 1979.

Part IV

Educational Communication

Chapter 7

Grant Getting

Carole J. Bland and Maureen M. Moo-Dodge

"I'm writing a grant proposal!" is a sentence fraught with hope and not a little hopelessness for most of us. In this chapter we plan to demystify many aspects of this task and in the process distill what we have learned both from our reading about grants and from our experience in writing, reviewing, and administering them.

First a word about words. Here are the definitions we are operating under: a *grant proposal* is your idea fleshed out in detail on paper. It is usually part of a larger work—the grant application. A *grant application* is a package of one or more proposals plus other information required by the agency from which you seek funds. A *grant* is money awarded.

The grant getting process builds like this: you develop an idea; you identify a potential funding source; you write a proposal about your idea; you prepare a complete application; you receive (in the best of all possible worlds) a grant award to carry out your idea. This order of activity is also the outline we follow in this chapter.

We assume that you, the reader, are either preparing a grant application yourself or are responsible for seeing that one is prepared. As we have already suggested, not only is that a multistage process, it also is a process calling for you to perform many functions. Probably none of us is equally effective at each of these functions. Thus throughout our discussion be alert to the proposal-writing or application-preparation functions that might or should be entrusted to a colleague with expertise in the area.

The actual writing of a grant application usually begins with drafting the proposal section. Several events, however, occur before you begin writing: Something or someone has stimulated you to consider this task, you have considered alternative funding mechanisms, and you have explored potential sources of support. Therefore, before focusing on how to prepare the proposal section of a grant application, we begin with a brief discussion of these preliminary events.

Getting Started

For family medicine faculty, at least four motivations prompt the considerable task of writing a grant proposal: personal interest, program needs, agency solicitations, and political and financial considerations.

Proposals often are written because someone wants to conduct research on a topic of enduring personal interest. For several reasons, a research proposal is perhaps the most rewarding type of proposal to write. It reflects the author's scholarly interests, its preparation generates a type of faculty renewal, and its completion produces a thoughtful contribution to the discipline.

Grant proposals also are written to garner support for training or service programs. Select funding agencies continue to earmark funds for family medicine programs. Therefore, family medicine faculty frequently write proposals seeking support to create, modify, or maintain a training program.

Proposals occasionally are written in response to an agency's solicitation. These proposals also may focus on research, service, or training needs, but in this instance they are prompted by an agency's specific request for proposals in a particular area.

Some proposals reflect political expedience. For example, when a funding agency requires evidence of interdisciplinary effort for a specific grant program, another department may ask your department to collaborate on their application. While doing so serves their needs, it simultaneously may benefit your family medicine department by building bridges to another department, raising an opportunity to co-author a proposal with an experienced grant writer, or introducing you to a funding agency you otherwise might not have contacted.

Whatever your motivation for wanting to write a grant proposal, before beginning, stop to ask yourself, "Is preparing a proposal the best way to accomplish this program or project?" This question really has two parts. First: Is a grant the best means of supporting the activity you want funded? Consider carefully other possible approaches. Perhaps your time would be better spent trying to secure patient-generated dollars, hospital support, or state appropriations. Grant awards have certain characteristics that may pose disadvantages for your purposes. Typically grants are given to projects or programs for which other funding is not available, they are competitively awarded, they are made for limited time periods—and they are growing smaller. If you are developing a permanent training program, for example, a grant might cover only start-up costs or provide funds to purchase one-time-cost items. Such a grant would not provide a stable way to fund ongoing costs such as faculty salaries or resident stipends.

Second: Can you prepare a lucid, persuasive proposal? Doing this means that you will be able to convince reviewers that an important problem exists and further that, having thoroughly researched the area, you now can propose an effective change. Do not underestimate the challenge of these tasks. Most granting agencies and funding programs require evidence that substantial planning has occurred on a project before they will invest in it. Even agencies that provide "seed" monies for development want to support projects that appear to have a head start, as shown by a thorough, clearly expressed proposal or by exceptionally qualified staff whose record speaks for itself. Demonstrating your planning ability is particularly important when you seek funds for a large or complex project. In this case, consider seeking financial support for several stages of the project: initially a needs assessment, then a pilot project, finally the large-scale project. You also might consider doing your project in conjunction with another project. If a colleague is writing a proposal or conducting a project in your area of interest, you might be able to accomplish your goals by joining forces, offering, for example, your expertise or patient population in return for using your colleague's resources.

Getting started then means seriously considering the appropriateness of grant seeking for your intended purpose.

Finding Out about Funding Sources

Once you decide that preparing a grant application is an appropriate means to seek funding for your program, you will move on to identifying potential funding sources. Should you approach internal or external funding sources?

Internal funding sources exist solely for the benefit of their parent institution, e.g., community hospital, professional organization, or university. Internal sources usually award modest amounts of money for 1-year projects that support activities such as curriculum development, research, travel, teaching or research assistance, or purchasing equipment. Grant announcements appear annually for the most part (though they sometimes appear on an irregular basis) and are sent primarily to deans, directors, or heads of agencies. In order to keep track of internal funding announcements, contact your institution's development office and arrange to be added to the mailing list. If that is not possible, arrange to have someone in the dean, director, or head's office send you a copy of the announcement. By keeping track of all internal grant programs for which you are eligible, even those whose deadline you may have missed that year, you will have a good idea of what is being offered and when. With a little investigating you also can discover what types of programs get funded and from this information judge whether or not your idea has a chance.

Major sources of external funding—foundations, the federal government and corporations—typically award larger sums for longer periods of time than do internal funding sources. When seeking external support you must meet specific eligibility requirements and show how your proposed project serves the specified goals and objectives of the funding agency.

Several excellent references can introduce you to external funding sources and describe the programs each offers. Brief descriptions of some of these reference tools follow. Although many more deserve mention, we selected the following sources because they are basic to any grant writer's library and because we think they will particularly interest grant seekers in family medicine.

Foundations

The *Foundation Directory*, compiled by the Foundation Center, describes over 3,000 foundations with entries organized by state. For each foundation the following information is given: foundation name, address, telephone number; purpose and activities; financial data, names of officers, trustees, or directors; and grant application information. Four indexes make this directory easy to use: Foundations; Foundations by State and City; Donors, Trustees, and Administrators; and Foundation Fields of Interest.

The Foundation Center also publishes several other reference tools to help grant seekers find the right funding agency; a few are listed below.

Source Book Profiles is a subscription service that presents information on giving patterns by subject area, type of support, and type of recipient for the 1,000 largest U.S. foundations.

Foundation Grants to Individuals describes grant opportunities for individuals. Most foundations do not award grants to individuals.

Foundation Grants Index Annual lists grant awards of $5,000 or more, briefly describes each, and reports recipient's name and location.

Federal Government

The Catalogue of Federal Domestic Assistance is a comprehensive listing and description of federal programs, projects, services, and activities available to the American public. Several indexes provide access to the mass of information collected in this catalog: Agency Program Index, Functional Index, Deadline Index, and Subject Index. Information for each program listed includes: name of federal agency administering the program, program authorization, goals and objectives of program, eligibility requirements, application and award process, examples of funding criteria, criteria for selection, financial information, and important telephone numbers.

The Federal Register is a daily publication announcing public regulations and legal notices issued by federal agenices. The section entitled "Proposed Rules and Regulations" provides details about proposed grant programs.

American Psychological Association Guide to Research Support provides detailed information about federal funding for research projects of interest to psychologists and other behavioral science professionals. For each of the 182 programs included in this guide the following information is given: description of the type of research supported, dollar amount available, description of past funding cycles including who received the award, amount of award, and duration of project; application procedures; and pertinent reference materials.

NIH Guide for Grants and Contracts announces research, training grants, and contracts supported by agencies of the National Institutes of Health. It provides policy and administrative information concerning opportunities, requirements, and changes in grants and contract activities to prospective grantees.

Corporations

The *Taft Corporate Directory* (1982) lists and describes corporate foundations. Indexes categorize the directory's entries by foundation name, state, field of interest, parent company, and type of grant made.

Individual annual reports provide an additional source—and one of the best—for information about corporate foundations and their grant making policies and procedures. To obtain an annual report, just call the development office or public relations office and ask for one.

Since corporate giving is highly localized, when you are looking for a corporate grantor look to your own community first. Remember that your proposal must be relevant to the corporation's business interests and usually it should have an impact on the corporation's employees, clients, or both. By examining the annual report, you will learn what the corporation is trying to accomplish through its giving program.

To sum up, three events typically occur before you start to write a grant proposal: (1) something has triggered your interest in writing a proposal; (2) you have decided that, among several possible funding mechanisms, a grant is an appropriate strategy to pursue; and (3) you have located a funding source likely to be interested in your project or program. Now preparing the actual proposal can begin.

Preparing a Proposal

The first step in preparing a proposal is to obtain the agency's guidelines, which should provide pertinent information such as the following:

Eligibility requirements

Due date (deadline)

Funding levels

Number of copies needed

Mailing address

Number of years for which support is available

Agency contact person and telephone number

Program goals

Review criteria

Date of award announcements

Carefully read the guidelines. Even if you previously have submitted an application to a particular funding agency, reread the guidelines. Agencies periodically make changes in guidelines and missing a changed requirement, for example, could jeopardize your application.

Foundations and federal agencies may request a letter of intent, also called a letter of inquiry, before you submit a formal proposal. The intent letter summarizes in two to four pages the rationale, goals, methodology, expected outcomes, and budget of your proposed project. After reviewing these letters, agency personnel either encourage you to submit a full proposal or advice you that your idea has little chance of receiving funding from their agency.

Besides their guidelines, some funding agencies provide application forms and budget sheets for you to complete. Most funding agencies, however, leave the structure of the proposal up to you, but request that you describe in detail your problem statement, objectives/hypothesis, strategies, evaluation, timeline, future funding, budget, and personnel.

When the agency does not specify a certain outline, one way of organizing your proposal is presented below, with a discussion of what belongs in each segment. Though the order may be varied, every proposal should include all the content described in each section (Krathwohl, 1977; Reif-Lehrer, 1982).

Introduction

Describe yourself or your program, emphasizing achievements to establish your credibility, and state the connection between your proposal and the goals of the funding agency.

Problem Statement

Define your problem and explain persuasively why something needs to be done.

The problem statement is the most important section of your proposal, for it induces the reviewer to read further. Here you must convince the reviewer that a significant problem exists or that information is lacking in the area that your proposal addresses. If you are unconvincing here, there is no reason for the reviewer to read on. For example, let us say that you are requesting renovation dollars for your family practice clinic under a residency training grant cycle. To defend the need for renovation you might present facts such as these: exam rooms currently available fail to meet basic criteria of number of rooms per resident; the entire facility is in disrepair (be specific—plaster cracks, warped flooring, etc.); remodeling is more cost effective than building or moving (present estimates for comparison).

Another example: Say you are seeking funds to investigate the effectiveness of caffeine elimination in the treatment of fibrocystic breast disease. Be sure to provide a concise but complete review of the literature applicable to your proposal. What other studies have looked at the effects of caffeine on breast disease? Is there important related literature such as the effects of alternative fibrocystic treatments? and so on. A good review assures readers of your competence in the area and enables them to understand the need for the study you are proposing. Since authors included in your literature review are likely to be among the people to review your application, it is especially important to demonstrate your comprehensive understanding of research already done in the area. Also, keep in mind that a literature review should report studies in an unbiased fashion. A reviewer could hold an opinion quite different from yours and this may color the review of your project.

Thus, whether seeking monies for training, service, or research programs, first you must be perfectly clear and persuasive about the need.

Objectives/Hypothesis

Clearly state what will be accomplished as a result of your project being funded. This means writing your objectives in a form that can be assessed or stating your hypothesis in a form that can be tested.

In a training or service proposal your proposal objectives should flow logically from your problem statement. In a research proposal the hypothesis for your study should flow logically from your literature review. Still, do not expect the reviewer to be able to reach your hypothesis or objectives simply from reading your background information. Instead, very clearly, with appropriate headings, state the hypothesis to be studied or the objectives to be accomplished if the proposal is funded.

Methods

If your proposal is organized by objectives rather than a research hypothesis, describe the strategies you will use to accomplish each objective. Be sure that the strategies you select are reasonable ones for accomplishing the objectives. If you select unusual strategies, justify why you have chosen them. For example, say you propose using drama groups to teach residents about the effects of alcohol abuse on the family. A drama group may be an effective teaching strategy for your program, its curriculum, and this problem, but the method will probably be unfamiliar to some of the reviewers.

If you propose a research study, be assured that it will be read by the most able scientists. Accordingly, in your methods section clearly identify the design and statistics to be used, perhaps displaying mock tables as an example of how data will be analyzed and summarized; discuss any problems you foresee in sampling and your plans to handle them; describe the validity and reliability of any measurement or data-collection instruments; and so on. In short, assure the reviewer that you have designed your study to yield accurate and useful data and have chosen the most appropriate strategies to analyze that data.

Evaluation

Both you and the funding agency will want to know if the objectives have been accomplished and whether the accomplishment of these objectives has helped to solve the identified problem. Thus, describe the evaluation methods you will use to assess the accomplishment of your objectives and the impact your project has had on the problem or question that initiated this proposal. Similarly, for a research proposal, prepare the reviewer for the results and conclusions you expect to draw with regard to your hypothesis.

Timeline

Provide a detailed, monthly timeline for the proposed project's first year. Specify what products you plan to produce and indicate when they will be completed. Record deadlines and activities with enough detail so that the reviewer will understand what you plan to do and will be convinced that you can do it. Allow yourself leeway in case some part of your project takes longer than expected. Do not overestimate or exaggerate the amount of work you can do in 1 year and, conversely, do not draw a project out to 3 to 5 years when it can be done in one. Be realistic in your time estimates. The reviewers will be. A general account of deadlines and activities is usually sufficient for the other years of the project.

Future Funding

Include a plan for continuing your activities (if appropriate) after the agency's funding is over. An agency is more disposed to fund an activity if you have made plans for continuing the project. Thus, if your research, training, or service efforts are intended to go on after the proposed budget period, seriously investigate how they will be financed and include your projections in your proposal. For example, the dean of your medical school may be willing to fund a course if, after 3 years of external funding, it has proved a valued part of the curriculum. Or perhaps, given 2 years lead time, you can plan to include the cost of the proposed project in your departmental budget.

The topics outlined above will guide you in completing a major portion of your application: the proposal section. Carrying out your proposed project will involve specific resources: salaries, training, research or service sites, or equipment. The next sections in the application center on presenting these financial details.

Preparing a Budget

Usually the budget for your project is described in two ways: a budget page and a budget justification. The budget page lists how much money is needed for specific categories: personnel, consultants, equipment, supplies, travel, etc. Funding agencies may provide a budget form for you to complete or you may be expected to devise your own. Table 7-1 presents an example of a typical budget page.

The budget justification describes why each item named on the budget page is needed and how the money will be spent. The largest budget category in most proposals is personnel. Accordingly, it is important that the budget justification for this category be clear, concise, and complete. Named first in this category is the project director or principle investigator. Ideally, this is the person who is masterminding and writing the proposal. Since this person is responsible for the content of the project, carefully plan and describe his or her time commitment and job responsibilities. If the director's responsibilities are incongruent with the time allotted to them, your proposal's credibility and the director's professed interest in the project are both suspect. Be sure that the salary figure presented is appropriate for a similar position at your institution.

Other personnel also help enhance your project's credibility. When you already have personnel who are particularly appropriate for your project, name them and include their qualifications and experience. If these individuals currently are employed full-time at your institution, explain how their job description would change as a result of the grant award. Assure the funding agency that the current levels of institutional support

Table 7-1. Budget Page: Psychosocial Medicine

A. Personnel

Name	Title of Position	Percentage of Time	Salary	Fringe Benefits	Total
C. P. Calhoun, M.D.	Project Director	75	$45,000	$10,800	$ 55,800
J. Nokomis, Ph.D	Coordinator	75	28,800	6,936	35,736
P. Hiawatha, Ph.D	Instructor	100	26,500	6,360	32,860
S. D. Cedar, Ph.D	Evaluator	50	14,000	3,360	17,360
W. Isles	Secretary	75	11,250	2,700	13,950
					$155,706

B. Consultants (including fee and travel)
Workshop I $450
Workshop II $3,310
    $ 3,760

C. Equipment—none requested $ - 0 -

D. Supplies
Photocopy $270   Brochure $520
Binding $135   Postage $400
    $ 1,325

E. Travel $ 2,400

    $163,191

will not be reduced or supplanted by a grant award. If you do not have a particular person in mind for a project position, it is still important to have thought about the type of professional that will be needed, including the person's credentials, job responsibilities, and time commitment. Your expectations in each of these areas should be written in the budget justification.

While we are on the subject of personnel and the budget justification, there is another companion bit of bookkeeping to be attended to here. Since it is easy to forget possible commitments made a year or more in advance, have all persons named in the personnel section document their intention to work on the project should it be funded. An easy way to accomplish this is to ask each person identified in the proposal to write a memo to the project director describing job responsibilities, time commitment, and salary. The faculty member also should specify the duration of his or her commitment to the project and should assure you that this time is available. In short, although you cannot totally commit someone to a proposal's anticipated activities, do be clear with each other about what is expected if the project is funded.

Getting back to the budget justification: other items commonly included in it are consultants, equipment and supplies, and/or travel. When justifying costs for the consultant category, whenever possible, name and describe the consultants. If you do not know whom you will be hiring, describe the type of person you will be looking for and what you want this person to do. Be as specific as you can about how long you expect the consultant contract to last and what you expect to pay the person(s) hired.

The equipment and supply categories should also be very specific. An explanation for an equipment request should include whether the equipment will be purchased or rented, type of equipment (model number, etc.), cost, who will use it, and who will maintain it. When addressing supplies, discuss what supplies will be needed and why.

Recently, the budget category of travel has received a great deal of scrutiny. Therefore, it is important to fully describe the reason for each trip, who will be making the trip (usually only one trip per major project personnel per year), how long each trip will last, and how much it will cost.

While not actually being a part of your budget, indirect costs contribute to the overall expense of your project. Indirect costs are a percentage of the total grant request or of only the personnel portion of it that is charged by your institution and are intended to cover expenses such as building rent, heat, maintenance, etc. Most institutions determine their own rate for indirect costs. Funding agencies, however, may or may not pay indirect costs, and if they do, they may determine their own rate. Thus, check with both the agency and your institution about indirect costs.

Do not underestimate the budget section's role in supporting the argument of your overall proposal. It is more than just numbers: it provides reviewers with important clues about how well the proposed project is thought out and how likely it is to be successfully executed. One last comment on the budget—be sure it adds up to the total you display on each and every budget page. Some reviewers love to check your math. Before mailing your application add your budget once more.

What Else Goes into a Grant Application?

So far we have discussed two parts of the proposal that comprise the core of your grant application: the highly persuasive proposal and its detailed accompanying budget. A grant application usually includes other information, both required and optional, which we describe next.

Letters of Affiliation

If your project includes other institutions or organizations, be sure to have a letter from each affiliate stating its agreement to cooperate as described in the proposal.

Letters of Support

Include letters of support from community agencies or prominent individuals addressing your ability to carry out the project successfully. Such letters perform three functions: They (1) influence reviewers' assessment of your ability to carry out the proposal, (2) assure reviewers of broad-based support, and (3) reinforce the need for your project.

Summary

You are wise to include a one- to two-page summary or abstract of your application. An abstract aids in both the initial reading of a proposal and the subsequent peer review process. Frequently, grants are reviewed in detail by two or more members of a larger peer review group. These primary reviewers prepare a summary of your grant that they present to the larger group for discussion and vote. The application that carries a summary written in the author's own words has an advantage over the one that requires a primary reviewer to construct a summary from his or her readings.

Before closing this discussion of the basic and "nice extras" sections in a grant application, we wish to mention two additional characteristics that should describe your proposal overall. While they are not discrete sections in a proposal, they deserve your attention because they can significantly bolster your credibility.

Personalization

Your proposal ought to sound as though a real person wrote it, not a nameless, faceless group. There should be signs that someone put heart and soul, as well as brain, into it. A reviewer is an impressionable reader after all. When, in addition to being well-organized, a proposal also has vitality and personal commitment throughout, a reviewer cannot help but react more positively toward it. And appropriately so, for if the proposal reflects an author who is already invested in the proposed project he or she will likely continue their efforts to assure success once funding is received.

Consistent Quality

Consistent quality—in writing style, in level of planning, and presentation format—also influences a reviewer's general attitude toward a grant. One weaker section or one larger incredulity in a proposal can make a reviewer doubt the whole. A reviewer inevitably forms an overall impression or attitude toward a grant. Consistently clear and believable writing throughout helps guarantee that the reaction will be positive.

Development Assistance from Agencies

While preparing your proposal you should establish and maintain contact with a program officer at the targeted funding agency. There are several legitimate questions you might ask to understand better what type of project the agency is likely to fund. Ask about the review process: What is the professional background of review panel members? What are the review criteria? If points are assigned to specific sections of a proposal, what section is worth the most points? Also find out about budget matters: What monies are available? Will the total be awarded proportionately by region? How many applications do they plan to fund? What is the estimated dollar amount per project? What have funding levels been in the past?

In addition, funding agency staff members can help you understand program guidelines and requirements and can provide advice on proposal outlines. If a grant program has been run several times, program officers often are aware of common mistakes and can give advice on how to avoid them. You also may be able to review previously funded grant applications. The federal government, for example, will send you past grants under the Freedom of Information Act. These requests must be made in writing, and you may be asked to pay for photocopying costs.

Agencies sometimes offer further special assistance. For instance, many large federal grant programs sponsor technical assistance workshops. Even if you have successfully competed in a cycle, attending these workshops is useful to assess the competition and to seek advice on how to improve your application. Use this time also to reestablish contact with your program officer.

Occasionally federal agencies and foundations will review preliminary proposals. More than a query letter or rough draft, a preliminary proposal should contain a well-thought-out need statement, goals, objectives, strategies, and evaluation. The budget should be developed in realistic detail. In many cases a preliminary proposal serves essentially the same purpose as a letter of inquiry: it forces you to organize your ideas, gives the funding agency a preview of your proposal, and allows them to give you an honest opinion about the match of your idea and the agency's goals. An agency's project personnel will be able to tell you whether or not a preliminary review is allowed. Since a preliminary proposal is a common strategy in proposal development, do not be shy about asking if this type of help is available. After you mail in your preliminary proposal, allow 2 to 3 weeks for review. When comments are offered, be ready to listen and be prepared to make changes. Do not argue. Reviewers are responding to what they understood. If they did not understand something as you intended it, you probably need to rewrite that portion of your proposal. Remember that since preliminary review is an informal process, written critique cannot be given.

Seek your colleagues' review of your proposal too. Peer review during the proposal writing process is an excellent way to get help on the content of your proposal.

It is as important after your application has been submitted as before to maintain contact with the agency. Though it is inappropriate to ask specific questions about how your proposal is being critiqued, you may appropriately ask the proposal's status in the review process and when you can expect notification of the agency's decision.

Developmental Assistance from Other Sources

You are seldom alone in proposal preparation. If you are in a fairly large program, department, hospital, or university, there are probably people nearby who have successfully prepared proposals, perhaps even for the agency to which you are applying. Seek out these people and their assistance. Some institutions also have developmental offices specifically to help their faculty prepare grant applications. If you have one at your institution, don't hesitate to inquire about its services for grant seekers. And, as already described, many funding agencies offer technical assistance to help you prepare a proposal according to their preferred style.

Submitting Your Application

When submitting your proposal follow the agency's guidelines exactly. Some major areas to be aware of are listed below.

Project Requirements

Often funding agencies specify project requirements that a proposal must meet before it will be reviewed. Sometimes elaborate, sometimes simple, in either case these requirements deserve your careful attention. An excellent proposal earns nothing if it is not reviewed because it failed to meet the requirements.

Page Limitations

Both federal and private agencies recently have begun to set application page limits. If your application exceeds size guidelines it might be returned to you unread.

Deadlines

Be sure to find out if the deadline refers to the postmark date or to the date an application must be in the agency's office. Send your proposals by registered mail.

Binding

Many agencies ask that proposals be paper clipped together, not stapled or bound. When the method of binding is specified follow the directions.

Organization

Remember, the person reviewing your proposal is probably already overworked, paid little or not at all for his or her peer review efforts, and reviewing numerous other applications. However the application is put together, be sure that the reviewer can easily locate information. At a minimum, furnish a table of contents. If your application is large, also separate each section with tabbed dividers. A reviewer who has to wade through pages and pages of narrative to find the problem statement, evaluation plan, and future funding section may take out his or her frustration in the review.

Number of Copies

Send the funding agency the required number of copies, making sure that one "master" copy contains all original signatures. Remember to make additional copies of the application for persons such as the project director and your institution's grant or development office.

Once You Are Funded

Federal agencies usually give grantees two to three months' notice before the funding starts. Local agencies may or may not give you advance notice. Once you are notified of funding, start preparing to execute the project and administer the budget. The following tasks specifically need to be completed before the project period starts.

Inform all personnel in writing that the project has been funded. Remind them of their responsibilities to the project, their time commitment, and their salary. If for any reason they must change any of these details, advise them to notify you as soon as possible.

Meet with project personnel and staff already on board to review each person's duties and responsibilities. Discuss procedures for advertising new positions, hiring new personnel, using travel dollars, buying equipment and supplies, and so forth.

Contact the grant administration office of your institution. Be sure that you understand how it will administer your budget, for example, if there will be any restricted funding categories. Also find out if project personnel will be required to account for their time and, if so, in what form will effort cards be circulated, for instance.

Know the name and telephone number of the person whom the granting agency has assigned as your project officer. Before the project begins, call to introduce yourself and ask any questions you have about the grant. Maintaining contact with the project officer is very important. Frequently a budget needs to be changed, an objective dropped, or the timeline altered. An informed and involved project officer can be extremely helpful when negotiating these changes with the funding agency. Even if changes are never needed keeping your project officer informed about a successful project will enhance your reputation as a reliable and capable project director. This is especially important when funding comes from a local foundation or corporation since these sources are more likely to be influenced by personal contacts.

Find out when progress reports and budget statements are due. Be on time and be thorough.

Remember, do not commit any money, spend any money, or hire anyone until the letter of payment has been received.

But If You Are Not Funded

When the unfortunate happens and you receive notification that your proposal was not funded, do not be discouraged. Experienced proposal writers will tell you that many of their grants are the products of two or three rejections, rewrites, and resubmissions.

If a federal agency turned down your application, the letter of notification will distinguish two possible reasons for rejection: either your application was approved but not funded, or it was disapproved. Approved but not funded means that, although reviewers recommended funding, the priority score they assigned it was not high enough for it to compete successfully against other applications for the funds available. When faced with this response, the project director should call the agency and request a copy of reviewer's comments.

At the federal level a proposal can be disapproved or rejected when reviewers determine that it does not fall within the agency's designated interest area(s) or it fails to meet the project requirements, or it cannot be accomplished for a variety of reasons (e.g., too ambitious, inappropriate budget, project director giving too little time or not being qualified, etc.). If your proposal is disapproved outright, again it is important to request reviewers' comments. They may contain suggestions that, if followed, would considerably strengthen your resubmitted proposal.

When preparing government grant applications you frequently work under deadlines that make it impossible to do as thorough a job as you would like. Therefore reviewers' comments can supply just the help needed to revise your proposal. A rewrite based on reviewers' comments often increases the application's priority score enough to secure funding from another source or from the original source during another funding cycle.

As for proposals rejected by a private foundation or corporation, it is appropriate to ask for reviewers' comments in this case as well. When no written reviewers' comments are available (often the case for small foundations and most corporate foundations), ask the agency's development officer for a critique of the proposal. Once again, rewriting your proposal according to the guidelines of this critique could result in a funded project next cycle.

To sum up: Grant getting requires a large and varied repertoire of skills. You must conceptualize like a scholar, argue like a successful barrister, arrange individual support like a seasoned politician, check adherence to requirements like an IRS pro, and prepare budgets with the steeliness of an accountant. Throughout you are an exemplary administrator merging the efforts of these varied activities into a highly integrated application. With appropriate time, resources, and interest, grant getting is also a manageable, stimulating, and enjoyable task that can have significant extrinsic rewards.

Faculty Development Activities

(1) Obtain a copy of an RFP (request for proposal) and the resultant grant. Review the RFP for stated requirements and purpose. Review grant for its ability to meet the requirements and for quality of proposed objectives/hypotheses.

(2) From a library or University Grants and Development Office obtain one or two directories of funding sources, e.g., *Foundation Directory*. Review these documents for variety of funding sources, and their funding preferences/goals.

(3) Identify the experienced grant writers in your institution or area. Set up an appointment with one of them and ask him/her to review the process they use to write grants.

References

Brownrigg WG. Effective corporate fundraising. New York: American Council for the Arts, 1982.

1982 Catalog of federal domestic assistance. Washington DC: Office of Management and Budget, 1982.

Federal register. Washington DC: Office of the Federal Register (daily).

The foundation grants index 1981. New York: The Foundation Center, 1982.

Foundation grants to individuals, ed 4. New York: The Foundation Center, 1982.

Foundation news. Washington DC: Council on Foundations, Inc. (bimonthly).

Henry R, Schoenthaler A, Grady S, eds: Taft corporate directory, 1982. Washington DC: Taft Corporation, 1982.

Krathwohl DR. How to prepare a research proposal, ed 2. Syracuse: Syracuse University, 1977.

The Grantsmanship Center news. Los Angeles: The Grantsmanship Center (six times per year).

Lewis MO, Gersumky AT, eds. Foundation directory, ed 8. New York: The Foundation Center, 1981.

Lowman RP, Holt VE, O'Bryant C, eds. American Psychological Association guide to research support. Washington DC: American Psychological Association, Inc., 1981.

Margolin JB: The individual's guide to grants. New York: Plenum Press, 1983.

Neilsen WA. The big foundations. New York: Columbia University Press, 1972.

NIH guide to grants and contracts. Bethesda, MD: National Institutes of Health, 1982.

Office of the Federal Register 1982–1983 United States government manual. Washington D.C.: Office of the Federal Register, 1982.

PanLener R, ed. Minnesota guidebook to state agency services, 1980–1981. St. Paul: Office of the State Register, 1980.

Reif-Lehrer L. Writing a successful grant application. Boston: Science Books International, Inc., 1982.

Smith CW, Skjei EW. Getting grants. New York: Harper & Row, 1980.
Source book profiles. New York: The Foundation Center (quarterly).
White VP. Grants: how to find out about them and what to do next. New York: Plenum Press, 1975.
White VP, ed. Grants that succeeded. New York: Plenum Press, 1982.

Chapter **8**

Curriculum and Instructional Applications

Katharine A. Munning

Introduction

As a teacher of family medicine, each faculty member has some responsibility for curriculum development and the instructional process. Components of this responsibility are overall design of the instructional system, development of integrated curriculum units (e.g., rotations, conference series, clinical continuity experience), preparation of educational objectives, participation in the instructional process, plus preparation of evaluation instruments and participation in the feedback process. Many books and articles describe the theory, importance, and processes of instructional design and curriculum development. This chapter will focus on the predominant writing skills required of faculty members to fulfill their educational responsibilities: writing educational objectives, instructional materials, and educational feedback/evaluation reports.

Instructional Objectives

Written instructional objectives contribute to the educational process in several ways. First, they provide direction for the teacher(s) and clearly communicate the educational intent to other instructors, or learners (residents, medical students, or others). Second, they provide guides for selecting content (e.g., type of patient population, conference topics), teaching strategies, and instructional materials. Third, they provide a guide for constructing evaluation instruments and the feedback process.

Therefore instructional objectives written as statements of learning outcomes are the cornerstone of the teaching/learning process. Figure 8-1 depicts this relationship. It is clear that learning experiences such as rotations, continuity experience, conference series, etc. are not ends in themselves but are tools to bring about desired learning outcomes. Also evaluation and feedback mechanisms are dependent upon clearly stated outcomes for their content and relevance to the final product.

Figure 8-1.   Relationships of objectives to instructional system.

Learner(s)

Resident
Medical student
Other health professionals

Teaching/Learning Process

Teaching strategies (examples):
  Rotations
  Conferences
  Patient care—episodic & continuous
  Journal club

Interaction of learner, content, teaching strategies, & instructional materials

General Learning Outcomes (End Products)

Knowledge/information
Problem solving skills
Communication skills
Technical/procedural skills
Professional attitudes and interests
Continuing education skills
Interpersonal/social skills

Evaluation System

Feedback in:

Achievement of learning outcomes
Effectiveness of teaching/learning process

In writing instructional objectives there are several general rules to follow:

(1) Begin each learning outcome with a verb that specifies definite, observable behavior.
(2) State each objective in terms of learner performance rather than teacher performance.
(3) Write each objective as a learning outcome rather than in terms of a learning process.
(4) State each objective so that it describes adequately the behavior of learners who have achieved the objective.
(5) Write each objective so that it includes only one learning outcome rather than a combination of several outcomes.
(6) Examine each objective for its relevance to the curriculum.
(7) Include complex objectives, e.g., clinical thinking, attitudes (even though they may be difficult to define in terms of specific behavioral outcomes).
(8) Consult reference materials to identify the specific types of behaviors that may be most appropriate for your complex instructional outcomes.

Avoiding Errors in Writing Instructional Objectives

One of the most common errors in writing objectives is to describe teacher behaviors rather than student behaviors. Of the two following statements which one most clearly indicates a learning outcome?

(1) Reviews journal articles for quality of research methodology.
(2) Increase the resident's ability to critically review the literature.

Obviously the first statement describes an expected outcome on the part of the resident. The second statement gives a less clear picture of the intended instruction of the teacher. It also inappropriately implies that the teacher will do the increasing rather than the resident.

The second common error in writing objectives is to state an objective in terms of a learning process rather than as a learning outcome. Verbs such as gains, acquires, develops give away the fact that an objective is written to focus on the process rather than the outcome of the learning experience.

A third common error in writing objectives is simply to list the various topic(s) to be covered in a curriculum unit. These are commonly seen as "laundry lists" of disease entities, diagnostic or therapeutic procedures, and concepts such as family dynamics or behavior modification. There is no indication of what a learner is expected to do with regard to the various topics listed. Is the resident simply required to define these terms, to understand them, or to be able to apply them in some particular situation?

Making lists of important content areas can certainly be the first step in
writing instructional objectives. The next step is to define the specific
behaviors we would want to observe in a resident managing a patient with
"congestive heart failure," performing a "pelvic exam," or understanding
the principles for "family dynamics."

Another common error is to choose a verb that is open to many
interpretations. A clear, precise, action verb is the key element in stating
specific learning outcomes. Table 8-1 contrasts global and specific verbs.

Writing Objectives Using the Taxonomy

The taxonomy provides a classification of instructional objectives that
encompasses all possible learning outcomes in hierarchial order from the
simplest behavioral outcomes to the most complex. The taxonomy is
divided into three parts: (1) the cognitive domain, (2) the affective domain,
and (3) the psychomotor domain. The cognitive domain includes those
objectives that emphasize intellectual outcomes such as knowledge,
understanding, and problem-solving skills. The affective domain includes
those objectives that emphasize feelings and emotion such as interest,
attitudes, and values. The psychomotor domain includes those objectives
that emphasize motor skills such as interviewing, physical exam, writing
SOAP notes.

This taxonomy system is based on the assumption that learning
outcomes can best be described in terms of changes in learner's behaviors.
Each domain is arranged in hierarchial order from the simplest behaviors
to the most complex. Each category is assumed to include the behavior at
the lower level(s).

Brief descriptions of the major categories in each of the three domains
are included in Tables 8-2, 8-3, and 8-4. Each table includes the major
categories in each domain, general instructional objectives, and specific
action verbs. The illustrative objectives are written in more global terms to
stimulate a broader range of specific objectives.

Table 8-1. Verbs—Global and Specific

Global (many interpretations)	Specific (few interpretations)
Know	Identify
Understand	Compare
Believe	Differentiate
Appreciate	Write
Learn	List
Gain an understanding	Solve
Grasp the meaning of	Strap
Become familiar with	Palpate

Table 8-2. Taxonomy of Objectives: Cognitive (Knowledge) Domain

Categories	General Objective	Specific Verbs
Knowledge	Knows medical terms Knows basic concepts, facts, and principles of basic and clinical sciences	Defines, lists, outlines, names, matches, states
Comprehension	Understands facts and concepts Interprets X-rays, EKGs, or other graphic material	Distinguishes, estimates, generalizes, infers, predicts explains
Application	Applies concepts, facts to new situations Demonstrates appropriate use of procedures, tests, etc.	Changes, computes, demonstrates, prepares, predicts, uses, solves
Analysis	Recognizes assumptions or logical fallacies in reasoning Distinguishes between fact and inference	Differentiates, selects, discriminates, identifies, outlines, infers
Synthesis	Proposes or writes a new plan Gives a well-organized conference	Categorizes, compiles, composes, explains, generates, revises
Evaluation	Judges adequacy of conclusions (chart audit) Judges value of a work by internal/external criteria	Appraises, compares, criticizes, justifies, concludes

The taxonomy should be used as a guideline to assist writers of educational objectives in drawing up a broad spectrum of learning outcomes including all three domains. It can also serve as a tool to clarify the specific level of required behaviors, especially for complex outcomes. Some objectives will include elements from all three domains. In summary, the taxonomy should serve as a guide for adequate listing of breadth of desired learning outcomes.

Instructional Materials

Faculty often use written materials as adjuncts to conferences, rotations, and other forms of instruction. Some of the commonly used written materials are bibliographies, lecture handouts of pertinent material, resident rotational manuals, protocols of medical care, and directions for performing a laboratory test or other manual procedures. In any of these applications, clarity, completeness, and helpful organization are of main importance. To achieve these outcomes, the writer must consider con-

Table 8-3. Taxonomy of Objectives: Affective (Attitudes) Domain

Categories	General Objective	Specific Verb
Receiving	Listens carefully Shows sensitivity to patients' needs Accepts cultural differences between patients	Asks, chooses, identifies, names, locates, selects
Responding	Completes patient encounter forms Obeys moonlighting rules Participates in residency committee	Answers, assists, conforms, writes, reports, discusses
Valuing	Demonstrates problem-solving attitude Shows concern for the welfare of patients	Completes, differentiates, explains, selects, shares, follows
Organization	Accepts responsibility for own behavior Understands and appreciates strengths and weaknesses Develops a life plan	Alters, defends, generalizes, compares, organizes, prepares
Value system	Maintains healthy life-style Practices cooperation in health care team Demonstrates responsible professional behaviors (e.g., punctuality, industry)	Discriminates, displays, influences, modifies, questions, reviews, verifies

stantly that instructions clear to an experienced family physician may not be clear to a resident or to a medical student. A first consideration therefore is always the reader of the instructional materials.

Knowing the Reader

Instructions that are to be used many times like resident manuals must be clear to all who use them, not just to the present residents. Words alone may not be enough; illustrations may be necessary. Complicated instructions, such as those for completing patient encounter forms or residency documentation cards, should be accompanied by a sample card or page. A model of the expected outcome is clearer than numerous descriptive paragraphs. If the learner is expected to differentiate the colors, shapes, etc., an illustration or sample of the desired outcome should be included in the instructional materials. A writer's first step in preparing these materials is to know the specific needs of the learners well enough to choose the words, illustrations, and samples required to present the topic clearly and concisely.

Table 8-4. Taxonomy of Objectives: Psychomotor Domain

Categories	General Objective	Specific Verbs
Perception	Recognizes malfunction by a sound or visual cue Relates a sign or symptom to an action	Chooses, detects, identifies, isolates, describes
Set	Knows sequence of steps Shows desire to learn skill	Begins, displays, moves, proceeds, reacts, volunteers
Guided response	Performs procedure as demonstrated Applies technique as demonstrated	Measures, tapes, sutures, organizes calibrates, sketches, constructs
Mechanism	Operates a piece of equipment Demonstrates a procedure or technique	(Same as guided)
Complex overt response	Operates equipment skillfully Demonstrates skillful and correct procedures	(Same as guided)
Adaptation	Adjusts or modifies technique to meet individual needs of patient	Adapts, alters, changes, rearranges, revises, varies
Origination	Designs a new method or technique Creates a new or improved procedure	Constructs, originates, arranges, combines

Knowing the Subject

The writer's second step is to be sure that he/she knows the subject completely. Thorough understanding of the topic or procedure may require that the writer actually experience it several times. Often, mistakes in directions/instructions come from a writer's failure to understand exactly what the learner will be asked to accomplish. For instance, it may be better to ask the head nurse on a ward rotation to outline required protocols, the billing clerk to describe the component parts of the patient encounter form, or the laboratory technician to describe the directions for doing a wet prep. A good writer uses the most reliable resources to assist in the task.

Organizing and Outlining

The third step is to outline instructions in the order of performance and to check the outline to be sure it includes all the steps or directions, listed in the correct order. A writer should not rely on a learner's reading all the directions before starting a rotation or performing a procedure. For this reason, any required equipment, supplies, references, or other necessary materials needed for the learning experience should be listed first.

Statements about safety should precede all other instructions. These safety instructions should be repeated just before any step where precautions are necessary. A writer should make it impossible for a learner to overlook a safety instruction by using a dramatic format (i.e., underlining words, color, large type) to highlight crucial information.

If a resident can follow the instructions more closely by understanding the rationale behind the instruction, then explanations should precede a set of directions or information. When sweeping changes occur in an instructional process such as a rotation, explanations are almost essential for residents to accept the new directions. A writer should always have a member of the intended audience (e.g., chief residents) read a rough draft or outline of a new set of directions and make necessary modifications. A justified, well-written manual of directions can help maintain the necessary structure in a multilocation, multifaculty resident training system.

Checking and Writing

Once an outline of necessary directions and/or instructions has been prepared, a writer should check it out by following the outline himself/ herself. The language of instructions and directions should be simple. Each step of the instructions should be in a new sentence and should be numbered. Illustrations should appear on the page or opposite page to which they apply and they should be legible enough that lettering or numbering can be read at a single glance. The directions for instructions should be so written as to indicate priorities. Unless the learner following the instructions or directions is so closely attuned to the writer that he automatically performs the tasks in the order desired, he is entitled to an indication of the appropriate order.

There is never any need to apologize for explicitness of directions, for the explanations or definitions that accompany them, or for a statement of order of performance. Directions that require an apology are those that are not explicit, clear, and organized.

Evaluation and Feedback Process

Evaluation is a crucial step in the instructional system. It provides information to teachers and students alike regarding achievement of desired outcomes and usefulness of chosen learning experiences. Many books and articles exist to help teachers write reliable and valid evaluation instruments. Therefore the following sections will focus on two areas of written skills not commonly found in the education literature.

Written Evaluation Reports

In family medicine we are asked to submit evaluation reports on individual learners or programs to faculties, funding agencies, and accreditation organizations. A formal evaluation report should be written similarly to a technical or research report. An outline of the content might be as follows:

(1) A front cover which provides the important identifying information about program, evaluators, period covered by the report, and date of report submission
(2) A summary overview of the evaluation
(3) Background information concerning the program to include goals, description of students, characteristics, and faculty
(4) Description of the evaluation study including purposes, design, outcome measures, implementation measures
(5) Results of outcome and implementation measures along with a discussion of informal results
(6) Discussion of results
(7) Costs and benefits (dollar and nondollar) including calculation method
(8) Conclusions and recommendations

An equally important component in the presentation of evaluation information is other written efforts to disseminate evaluation information through memos, news releases, and any other written communication. Several tips for using the written medium to communicate evaluation information are:

(1) Start with the most important information. When reading for information, readers tend to seek out the most important points first; therefore, the opening paragraph or section should specify the principal message.
    A rule of conciseness is to "imagine that your reader will not have time to get through the whole report." Plan that some interruptions will cause the report to be laid aside and not picked up again. Choose your words carefully and say it right away. As much as possible start each chapter, subsection, or paragraph with the most important point you wish to make in that section.
(2) Highlight the important points by the following methods:
    (a) Use descriptive subheadings;
    (b) Try using headings as a running commentary to the left and parallel of the report text;
    (c) Space and lay out the report text to highlight important information such as: using an outline format with more white space, boxing in important information to highlight; *making changes in type set*; underlining; or using CAPITAL LETTERS.

(3) Make your report readable:
  (a) Create an image of the intended reader and describe this person. As you write keep this individual in mind;
  (b) Use familiar words, not jargon;
  (c) Use action verbs as much as possible;
  (d) Cut out dead wood such as unnecessary words and phrases;
  (e) Shorten your sentences and paragraphs;
  (f) Try a personalized style to include first-person pronouns, contractions, and, when appropriate, "shirtsleeve" language.

Writing Feedback

One of our most important functions as teachers is to provide constructive, balanced feedback to our residents and medical students. Feedback often occurs in both oral and written mediums. Written feedback is commonly seen in chart audits, periodic summaries of a resident's performance, open-ended statements on family medicine rotation evaluations, and letters of recommendation. Table 8-5 describes the characteristics of balanced feedback, which are the same for both oral and written. Information contained in the written statement needs to be behavior specific and free of misinterpretation. It is helpful to describe the method by which the descriptive information was gathered (e.g., direct observation, chart audit), your relationship to the individual and the use of this information in the evaluation system.

The style used in writing the feedback should be specific to the situation and the individual(s) reading the written statement (i.e., resident, other faculty, nonfamily medicine faculty, etc.). Once you have analyzed the situation and the cast of characters, there are several questions to be answered.

Do you want to be personal and warm? Usually yes, but in this situation?

Do you want to communicate clearly and directly and forcefully? Usually yes, but here?

Table 8-5.   Characteristics of Balanced Feedback

(1) Descriptive rather than judgmental
(2) Specific rather than general
(3) Focused on behavior rather than on the person
(4) Solicited rather than imposed
(5) Well timed
(6) Concerns what is "said and done," not why
(7) Takes into account needs of both receiver and giver of feedback
(8) Discussed to assure clear communication
(9) Contains positive feedback as well as suggestions for change

Do you want to seem to be downplaying the conflict or negative situation?

Do you want to approach the issue with a great deal of information, or passively?

What is the strategically appropriate style? The choice of style is a matter of judgment by the faculty member in a given situation. Judging the situation and the reader of the written feedback accurately separates successful written feedback from unsuccessful.

Forceful Style

A forceful style is most appropriate in situations where the writer has power and influence and wants to communicate a directive.

(a) Use the active voice ("correct this error immediately" rather than "a correction should be made").
(b) Be clear and direct. Do not beat around the bush ("I have decided not to approve your moonlighting request" instead of "Unfortunately a positive recommendation for your moonlighting request is not forthcoming").
(c) Write most of your sentences in a subject/verb/object order. Do not weaken them by putting in phrases before the subject.
(d) Do not weaken sentences by relegating the point of action. ("Dr. Jones did a superb job on the rotation, although the patient volume was low" not "Although Dr. Jones did a superb job the patient volume was low on the rotation").

Passive Style

This style is often appropriate in negative situations, when the writer is in a lower position than the reader, or when the writer does not have a trust relationship with the reader. It can be used in distant situations where there is no opportunity to discuss the content.

(a) Avoid the imperative. Never give an order.
(b) Use the passive voice heavily because it subordinates the subject to the end of the sentence or buries the subject entirely. The passive voice is especially important when you need to convey negative information to a reader who is in a higher position than yourself. ("Valuable sources of patient revenue are being wasted" instead of "you are under-charging your patients.")
(c) Avoid taking responsibility for negative statements by attributing them to faceless, impersonal others. ("The evaluations show that" rather than "Our chief residents have said.")
(d) Use long sentences and heavy paragraphs to slow down the reader's comprehension of the sensitive or negative information.

Personal Style

This style is especially appropriate in good news and persuasive situations. It displays and builds relationships.

(a) Use the active voice, which puts you as the writer at the front of the sentence. ("Thank you very much for your comments" or "I appreciated comments" rather than "your comments were very much appreciated by me" or more impersonally, "your comments were very much appreciated.")
(b) Use persons' names—first names when appropriate—instead of referring to them by title.
(c) Use personal pronouns, especially you and I, when you are stating positive things.
(d) Use short sentences that capture the rhythm of ordinary conversation.
(e) Use contractions to sound informal and conversational.
(f) Direct questions to the reader.
(g) Interject positive personal thoughts and references that will make the reader know this letter is meant for him/her and is not a form letter.

Impersonal Style

This style is usually appropriate in situations in which you wish to convey information or data, such as technical and scientific reports.

(a) Avoid using a person's name.
(b) Avoid using personal pronouns, especially you and I.
(c) Use the passive voice to make yourself conveniently disappear.
(d) Make some of your sentences complex and some paragraphs long. Avoid the brisk, direct simple sentence structure of conversation.

Obviously these styles are not mutually exclusive. Before making a choice, decide which is most appropriate given the content of the feedback, your relationship with the reader(s), and the purposes for which the document was written. Since negative information is especially difficult to convey, it may be important to reinforce written information with oral clarification and discussion. Therefore, determine ahead of time what information you will need to discuss personally with the reader to assure communication of the written word and clarification of information.

Faculty Development Activities

(1) Make a list of topics you think are important in Family Medicine (e.g., family dynamics, prenatal care, health maintenance). Choose one

topic and write at least five cognitive, five psychomotor, and five affective objectives. Be sure and use the verb lists included in the chapter.

(2) Assemble the educational objectives used in your residency program. Review these objectives for the presence of an action verb, specific behavioral descriptions, and learner orientation.

(3) Audio or videotape one of your precepting encounters with a resident or medical student. Listen to the tape and write the learning objectives based on the content of that encounter. To provide the best care for that patient, what knowledge, skills, and attitudes would you want the resident to possess?

(4) Using the taped precepting encounter, practice writing balanced, behavior-specific feedback you would like to give the resident.

(5) Include balanced, behavior-specific feedback in your next chart audits. Choose the appropriate style.

References

Fabb WE, Heffernan MW, Phillips WA, Stone P. Focus on learning in family practice. Melbourne: Royal Australian College of General Practitioners, 1976.

Fielden JS. What do you mean you don't like my style? Harvard Business Review, May–June 1982;128–38.

Gagne RM, Briggs LJ. Principles of instructional design. New York: Holt, Rinehart and Winston, 1979.

Gronlund NE. Stating objectives for classroom instruction. New York: Macmillan Publishing Co. Inc., 1978.

Holcombe MW, Stein JK. Writing for decision makers. Belmont, California: Lifetime Learning Publications, 1981.

Kibler RJ, Cegala DJ, Watson KW, Barker LL, Miles DT. Objectives for instruction and evaluation. Boston: Allyn and Bain, 1981.

Mager RF. Preparing instructional objectives. Belmont, California: Fearon Publications, 1975.

McKeachie WJ. Teaching tips: a guidebook for the beginning college teacher. Lexington, Mass.: DC Heath and Co., 1978.

Mills GH, Walter JA. Technical writing. New York: Holt, Rinehart and Winston, 1978.

Morris LL, Fitz-Gibbon GT. How to present an evaluation report. Beverly Hills: Sage Publications, 1978.

Chapter **9**

Writing Patient Education Materials

Don W. Bradley and Bruce F. Currie

In an age of increasing public awareness about health-related issues, the concept of patient education is increasingly important. Patients expect and demand better information from health care providers, as well as from various media. Through patient education, the medical profession has an opportunity to improve provider–patient relationships and to enhance medical care.

This chapter is designed for those who both educate patients and are responsible for teaching patient education skills to health care providers and office staff. Only written skills in patient education are covered, but many of these skills can be generalized to all forms of patient education. Upon completion of this chapter, the reader should be able to:

(1) define patient education,
(2) describe the advantages and limitations of written materials in patient education,
(3) list and discuss five major areas to consider when designing patient education materials (practicality/implementation, relevance/acceptability, content, format, and effectiveness/evaluation),
(4) evaluate a patient education handout using the instruction provided,
(5) given the evaluation, suggest changes to improve its effectiveness.

Definition of Patient Education

Patient Education is the process among the patient, patient's family/support system, and the provider of:

(1) mutually understanding the significance and implications of the patient's symptoms and/or
(2) mutually agreeing on the importance of a health promotion behavior; and
(3) then developing a plan which the patient can reasonably follow to improve or maintain health.

Communication in all forms, including written material, is the backbone of patient education. Although written materials alone cannot fulfill the definition, they can be a potent aid in accomplishing patient education goals.

In this chapter, most emphasis will be placed on printed materials prepared commercially or in the provider's office. However, handwritten notes, stickers, or labels also qualify as written communications. Their uses, although more limited, are nevertheless important, and follow the same principles as those for printed instructions.

Advantages and Limitations

Instructional handouts have been shown to be highly valued by patients, and effective in increasing their knowledge and compliance (Gadd et al., 1981; Morris and Halperin, 1979). The same reviews, however, indicate that the written word is not necessarily the best method of communication. Multiple forms of communication, especially verbal and written instructions used together, are even more effective in transferring knowledge and channeling behavior. These studies bear out the intuitive notion of many family physicians that the patient handout is best used as an extension, rather than a substitute, for the office visit. Written materials are most effective when used to reinforce instructions previously discussed by the provider.

Flexibility, convenience, and the ability to transmit or reiterate knowledge are the primary advantages of the printed medium. Its limitations relate mostly to the patient's ability to *read*, and the lack of person to person contact. A detailed summary of the pro and con factors of printed materials is shown in Table 9-1. They can be used to decide whether such materials can help with a given problem.

Considerations in Writing Patient Education Materials

When the advantages of a written handout outweigh its limitations, the next step is the process of planning a patient education module. The following five considerations serve both as a guide to writing and as an evaluation tool for already prepared materials. Each area will be discussed briefly, and then strategies will be suggested to deal with the problems encountered.

Table 9-1. Advantages and Limitations of Written Materials

Advantages	Limitations
(1) Patients can learn at their own pace	(1) Patient must be able to read and understand handout
(2) Can be adapted to different languages or reading levels	(2) Is not interactive—no immediate feedback
(3) Offers another learning strategy as a patient	(3) Many commercial materials are not suitable for physician's practice style
(4) Can be customized for the individual	(4) Commercial materials can be overly expensive
(5) Can be used to transfer larger quantities of information than is possible by verbal communications	(5) Providers must allocate time to prepare or review materials
(6) Ready-made materials are frequently available	
(7) Can be produced on-site	
(8) Can be available in varied locations (waiting room, exam room, mailings, etc.)	
(9) Can be reproduced inexpensively on copy machine	
(10) Easily portable	

Feasibility/Practicality

The first question that arises is that of redundancy—with the plethora of materials already available, should new handouts be prepared? Except for a simple handwritten note, most materials take several hours to develop and write. To reproduce them takes more time and money. Also, most office settings have only limited capabilities to illustrate, format, and print such materials.

Another important practical consideration is when and how often the handouts will be used. Many practices have accumulated an impressive collection of patient handouts from multiple sources, but most of them remain unused. Often, handouts pertain to problems rarely encountered in normal clinical settings. (For instance, there is little use for a beautifully written pamphlet on Zollinger–Ellison Syndrome.) The patient education file can become so crowded with extraneous material that even the most dedicated patient educator cannot or will not use the handouts. A large file also requires time and expense to evaluate and keep current.

Strategies

A very practical approach is to choose the 10–20 most common problems the practitioner faces. In the Duke–Watts Residency, common problems include hypertension, upper respiratory tract infections (URI), prenatal care, diabetes, cystitis, otitis media, obesity, and depression. Some problems may require more than one handout. For example, both an explanation of URI and a sheet to explain fever control are helpful.

There are several resources for "freebies" such as the drug companies, community health agencies, and in some areas, hospitals. There are also several excellent compendiums of patient education materials (Brunworth and Rigden, 1979; Griffith, 1975, 1978, 1980; McCormick and Gilson-Parkevich, 1979) as well as individual commercial handouts. If the prepared form fits your practice and philosophy, use it. If not, modify it, or use it as a model for your own handout.

When you do need to develop your own materials, write short (one to two pages), simple handouts. Several authors may collaborate on one handout—physicians, patient educators, office staff, nurses, students, and/ or patients. Each provides a unique perspective, and joint efforts sometimes lessen the cost and time required of the provider.

Relevance/Acceptability

Even though producing a handout is worth the provider's time and effort, will it be useful to the patient? Are patients interested in what providers have to say? Are they able to integrate the information, and will they believe and act upon it?

Health care providers often assume that patients are interested in their comments simply because the patients present themselves to the office. What patients want or need, however, is not always easy to discern. If a patient comes in with low back pain, but really wants to talk about his/her depression, no amount of education about back pain is likely to help. The patient may have come to talk, not to read. Barsky (1981) points out patients' hidden reasons for visiting a doctor, such as their needs to feel cared for, as well as needs for information about symptoms. In the above example, the patient's expectation may be a prescription for pain medicine. A well-written and presented pamphlet, however, may better fulfill the patient's real needs for reassurance and sense of appropriate provider concern. The pamphlet, used in place of the prescription, not only avoids the use of medications but also gives the patient new knowledge and strategies to deal with the discomfort.

The Maslow Model

To decide what is relevant and acceptable to your patients, consider the following model that describes patient needs. Maslow's theory of human motivation describes a hierarchy of human needs. He believed that the most basic or survival needs must be met before higher needs can be pursued (Chatham and Knapp, 1982) (see Figure 9-1). Survival needs in Maslow's schema would include the physiological necessities—food, clothing, shelter, and sleep. In terms of medical care, the same needs exist, but also included are emergency problems—how to stop a bleeding artery, how to take nitroglycerin when angina begins, the phone number for an ambulance or doctor's office in an emergency, etc.

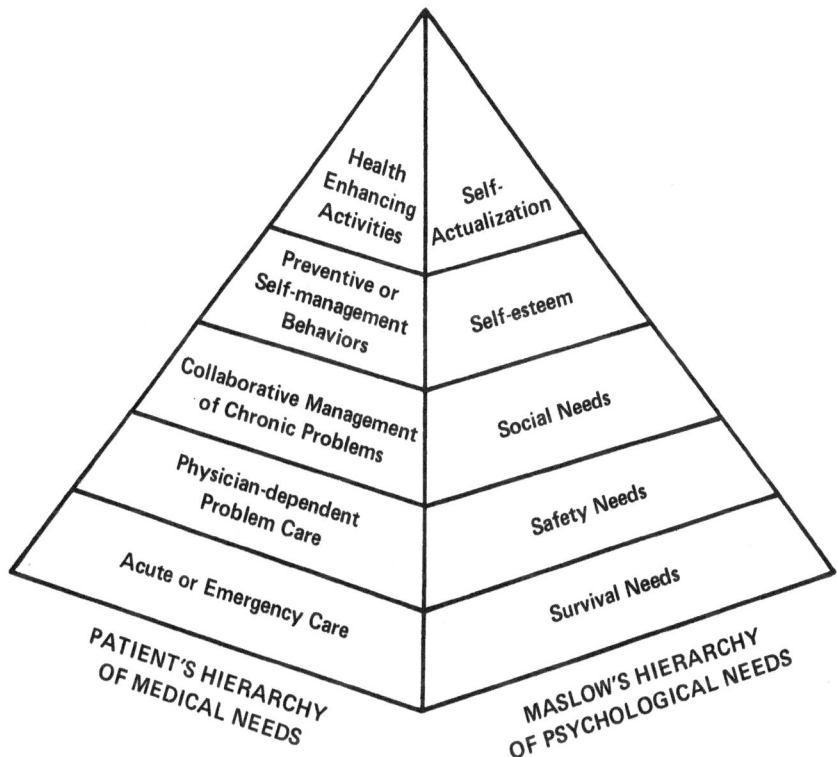

Figure 9-1   Patient needs important in writing patient education materials.

Safety needs, such as job security, finding the way around town, or feeling safe in the home, are a second level of the hierarchy. Many of the patient's safety needs are also provided by the physician—how to take daily medicine, what side effects of treatments can be expected, what activities are allowed, rudimentary explanations of pathophysiology, etc.

The next level on the pyramid entails social interactions, like making friends and finding people with similar interests. The patient begins to ask questions and contribute suggestions for the treatment plan. The effect of the family is considered. For example, Mr. Jones may ask if he can take his blood pressure medicine twice a day rather than four times a day, to better suit his schedule. His wife may be inclined to reinforce his low salt diet.

Further up the hierarchy, self-esteem needs emerge, such as feeling good about oneself in general and feeling that one's contribution to family and friends is worthwhile. In medical terms, the patient develops the skills and confidence for self-management and preventive behaviors. Examples are home monitoring of blood pressure, adjusting insulin dose to match diabetic urines, and exercise and walking programs.

Finally, there is nirvana—self-actualization—where the individual is comfortable with his/her own accomplishments, and accepts personal strengths and weaknesses. In a medical sense, the patient participates in health enhancing behaviors for the sake of feeling good, not to avoid or manage a problem.

The level of the patient education material must fit the level of the patient's needs. For instance, patients who have an acute myocardial infarction or who are under a great deal of emotional or physical stress are unlikely to absorb much information about detailed physiology or management. Many materials deal only with social and self-esteem needs, and are far too advanced for patients at lower need levels in the hierarchy.

Strategies

Decide for what group of patients you are writing and match their educational and interest levels. Include the basics first—a lay title for the problem, how to treat it, and when to come back. If there is time, room, and interest, progress up the hierarchy of needs. Remember the handout is written to meet the patient's needs, not the provider's. Two or three handouts may be needed for the same problem one for basics and a more detailed handout suited to advanced interests. For diabetic patients, consider providing an initial folder of printed materials, that gives the survival steps—how to inject insulin, when, how much, etc. More complicated materials can be added as the patient assimilates the basic information.

Content

The content of written communication is crucial. Without the message, there is no need to write. Too often, however, consideration of content focuses solely on whether information is medically correct and current. Certainly accurate, up-to-date data are important, but can be lost in content "traps."

The first trap is presenting too much information to the patient. Overenthusiastic to "educate," providers sometimes present pages of explanations and treatment plans, only to lose the most important points in the flood of information. A general rule of thumb is to present only five to seven points at a given time. Beyond that number, patients either forget or lose interest. Written communication does allow for greater transfer of information, since patients generally remember only three to four important points from verbal encounters.

The second trap is writing far above most patients' reading levels. Doak and Doak (1980) discovered that most patients' reading comprehension levels are at the seventh and eighth levels. Most patient education materials are written at a tenth to twelfth grade level. The reading level of most patients is two to four grade levels below the number of years of school finished. Thus, a patient requires at least a high school diploma and a year or two of college to read most patient education materials. (This chapter, incidentally, is written at a fifteenth grade reading level.)

The third trap is lack of specificity and practicality. Even when the patient is presented with a limited amount of materials at an appropriate level, the material needs to be practical and specific. Often a written handout tells the patient to call the doctor for problems, yet fails to provide a current phone number. Or, it will instruct a patient to take a medication without noting how much or when. Although medical personnel are quite accustomed to medical routines and terminology, the patient is dealing with a new language and set of rules.

The fourth trap is transmitting messages not meant to be sent. Patients interpret quite literally. If they read, "the fever *must* be brought to normal," a sense of urgency is implied. Will the patient die or be permanently damaged if the fever is not brought down, or will he/she merely be uncomfortable? Terms such as "always," "must," and "never" can some-times convey unwanted, unsuspected messages.

The final trap is writing in an unnecessarily complicated style. Con-voluted sentences are as difficult to understand as misspelled words. A recent patient education pamphlet about Reye's syndrome (HHS Publica-tion No. (FDA) 82-3126) explains, "Therefore, the Food and Drug Administration, an agency of the Public Health Service, has proposed that aspirin and other salicylates, and medications containing aspirin, be labeled with a warning against giving them to children under age 16 with influenza, chicken pox (varicella) or other flu-like illnesses." The sentence delivers an important message, simply stated, "Children under age 16 should not take aspirin products for 'flu' or chicken pox." The second sentence is much clearer than the first.

Strategies

Review what has been written by others. The content may not fit your practice situation or philosophy, but it is starting point. Label controversies as such. The patient will be confused if he/she receives contrary information. List the five to seven most important points you want your patient to remember. Then write the handout. It may be helpful to have someone else read your handout, especially a patient. If this patient sees different or more important points, then the message is not clear enough.

Test the reading level of your materials using the SMOG Readability (McLaughlin, 1969) formula:

(1) Count off 10 consecutive sentences near the beginning, in the middle, and near the end of the handout.

(2) In this sample of 30 sentences, circle all the words containing 3 or more syllables, and total them.
(3) Take the square root of the nearest perfect square to the total number (i.e., if you counted 69 polysyllabic words, the nearest perfect square is 64, and the square root is 8).
(4) Add a constant of 3 to the square root—this is the reading level (grade).

To test a handout with fewer than 30 sentences, use the following formula:

(1) Count all the polysyllabic words and count all the sentences.
(2) Divide the number of sentences into 30. (If 15 sentences—30/15 = 2).
(3) Multiply the number of polysyllabic words by the number obtained in step 2.
(4) Find the square root of the nearest perfect square to the number in step 3.
(5) Add a constant of 3 to obtain the reading level (grade).

Match this reading level to your usual patient panel. Remember that patients will probably need to have finished two to three more years of school to read at this level.

Another approach is to write all patient education materials at the seventh to eighth grade level, assuming that most patients read at this level. In writing for lower reading levels, shorten sentences, use common words, and replace polysyllabic words with one- or two-syllable words. A conversational style helps comprehension, and conveys a more personal message.

To allow for practical information, leave space to hand-individualize handouts. Medicines doses, times, phone numbers, and return appointment dates can be jotted in by you or the patient during the encounter.

Format

The purpose of the handout's format is twofold. First, it interests the reader in what is written. Second, it helps the reader organize and understand the material.

Written patient education materials come in all sizes, shapes, colors, and prints, each with its own merits. Especially for materials produced in the office, print and illustrations should be simple. Large and adequately spaced print is easier to understand and easier to see (think of elderly or visually handicapped patients). Illustrations are useful, and need not be sophisticated. Patients prefer realistic pictures, but crude drawings are as effective in helping patients learn (Levie, 1973). McCormick and Gilson-Parkevich (1979) provide an excellent discussion that extends far beyond the scope of this chapter.

Strategies

Keep it simple. Use 8½ ×11 in. paper (it is cheaper, easier to store, and allows a great deal of flexibility). Use clear, large print with adequate spacing. Emphasize major points with boldface type or underlining. Try to present major points early in the handout.

Use illustrations to clarify points of anatomy or procedures, or graphs to emphasize major points. Graphs or tables best summarize important information, and color attracts attention or differentiates topics clearly.

Effectiveness

The effectivenss of written patient education materials depends both on the quality of the handout and the way it is used in the total practice. If written handouts are a new, nonintegrated activity, then they are not likely to meet with much success. The attitude of the office staff, the office floor plan, and patient flow all need to be part of an integrated, organized patient education system.

Proving effectiveness is difficult. Studies have tried to correlate effectiveness with measures of patient satisfaction, patient knowledge, medication compliance, and overall health. The ultimate outcome, a healthful change in patient behavior, is affected by multiple factors. Recent research presents contradictory conclusions but is optimistic. The Time—Seagram study (Schiller et al., 1982), for instance, demonstrates that changing attitudes is not a prerequisite for changing behavior. The implication for patient education is that measurements of effectiveness should include outcome behaviors rather than "intermediate" steps such as changes in attitudes. More study is needed in this area.

Strategies

Ask your child, your office staff and friends to read your patient education materials. If they understand (and like them), at least the barriers of relevance and comprehension are out of the way.

Evaluate your materials before you give them to patients—know what each handout says. Use handouts as an extension of the office visit.

Keep handouts in convenient, accessible locations—the waiting room, the exam room, etc.

Putting It All Together

Using the five considerations for writing patient education materials, the reader should now be able to write and/or evaluate any given handout. Table 9-2 depicts a handout from the Duke–Watts patient education file. Using the evaluation instrument (Table 9-3) to rate this handout is a useful

Table 9-2. Upper Respiratory Tract Infection ("Cold")

Epidemiology: Upper Respiratory Tract Infection (URI) or "colds" are caused by one of several viruses, are more common in the winter months, and are spread by droplet transmission. Most URI's last 3–7 days, and since many different viruses can cause the infection, people can have several colds in a row, each caused by a different virus.

Anatomy and physiology: Colds cause inflammation of the nose, throat, eustachian tubes, sinuses, trachea, and bronchial tubes. The symptoms created include stuffy nose, sore throat, dry cough, fatigue, malaise, and fever. The worst symptoms of congestion usually occur on the third and fourth days. The cough may last up to 6 weeks, but should decrease gradually with time.

Treatment:
(1) Rest—if the patient has a significant fever (greater than 101°F or 38°C), he/she should be kept quiet indoors. If there is no significant fever, activity as tolerated is permissible. Children should be kept home from school if the fever is greater than 101°F.
(2) Fluids—Drink plenty of fluids. Solid foods are not essential, and are not very appetizing to most patients during a cold.
(3) Medications and Treatment
    (a) Antibiotics generally are *not indicated* since viruses will not respond to them—most medicines are meant only to relieve symptoms, not to cure the infection.
    (b) A cool mist vaporizer placed next to the patient's bed will often relieve congestion. Decongestants may also be helpful.
    (c) Cough medications—Any cough syrup with dextromethorphan will help. Be sure not to take two similar medications, since overdosing may occur.
    (d) Fever—Aspirin or Acetaminophen—keep the fever less than 102°F for comfort (see fever sheet).
Call your doctor if:
(1) the temperature cannot be lowered below 101°F, for shaking chills, or if fever persists for more than 2–3 days.
(2) the primary symptom is sore throat without runny nose, cough, etc.
(3) sputum turns yellow or green, or contains blood
(4) increasing shortness of breath, wheezing, or cyanosis
(5) increasing lethargy, irritability
(6) inability to keep down sufficient fluids.
Prevention of URI's:
(1) Cover the mouth when coughing or sneezing.
(2) Use separate eating and drinking utensils.
(3) Avoid crowded places and close contact with people with colds.

exercise to train you to evaluate materials produced inside and outside your own practice. The highest score possible is "60." The absolute score is not as important as the ability to compare different handouts.

Using the evaluation instrument, note that the handout covers the common cold, an upper respiratory tract infection. The problem is commonly seen in most practices, and the handout inexpensive to produce. It is designed to cover all aspects of a URI, including prevention. Some specifics are available for basic needs, such as how long the patient needs to stay home.

But the handout fails to say which medicines should be taken, how much, and when. The attempts at providing midlevel knowledge, such as anatomy and physiology, are clouded by highly technical terms—eustachian tube, trachea, URI, etc. The major points are highlighted by headings, but there are too many points under each subtitle. There are three points under "Treatment," six points under "Call Your Doctor If," and three points under "Intervention."

The medical content is current and accurate, and seems mildly helpful. Again, what medicines should the patient take? The print is readable, if crowded. Headings are used moderately well to organize the handout. There are no illustrations. The major points are not well delineated. No attempt is made to individualize the form.

The reading level is the eleventh grade—(24 sentences, 50 polysyllabic words $(30/24 \times 50) = 62.5$. The nearest square is 64, its square root is 8. Add the constant of 3, $8 + 3 = 11$).

Overall, the effectiveness of this handout in our practice is poor to fair. This handout rates about 35.

Given the suggestions above, the "Cold" handout was rewritten, (see Table 9-4). The new handout is more eye catching, useful, and certainly easier to read. Using the evaluation instrument again, the redone handout rates a 53 out of 60.

Conclusion

Written patient education materials can be effective, time-saving aids in most medical practices. This chapter discusses practical strategies to make handouts useful and cost effective. An evaluation instrument is provided to judge which handouts are most helpful.

Faculty Development Activities

(1) Outline your personal philosophy about patient education. Share with your colleagues and determine program's philosophy.
(2) Using Maslow's Need Theory, outline the content for a patient education document/handout.

Table 9-3 Evaluation Form

Patient Education Handout						
Title: _____						(1)
Problem/Topic: _____						(2)
Source: _____						(3)
Date produced: _____ ___ / ___ / ___						(4)
Reviewer: _____ ___ ___ ___						(5)
	Unacceptable	Poor	Fair	Good	Excellent	
Feasibility—Cost _____	1	2	3	4	5	(6)
Frequency of Problem Covered	1	2	3	4	5	(7)
Relevance/Acceptability—[Designed for: 1=self-motivated health behaviors, or 2=prevention & self management, 3=social—patient & family collaboration, 4=safety/more detailed instructions, 5=survival—only the basics]	1	2	3	4	5	(8)
Content—List 5 major points covered: 1. 4. 2. 5. 3.						
Overall clarity of points	1	2	3	4	5	(9)
Medical content is accurate & current	1	2	3	4	5	(10)
Content is practical and useful	1	2	3	4	5	(11)
Reading level (SMOG) ___ grade <1=12+, 2=10−12, 3=8−10, 4=6−8, 5=<6)	1	2	3	4	5	(12)
Format—Print is readible, adequate subtitles	1	2	3	4	5	(13)
Illustrations pertinent, clear	1	2	3	4	5	(14)
Major points are emphasized by format (underlines, presented early, summarized)	1	2	3	4	5	(15)
Room for individualization	1	2	3	4	5	(16)
Effectiveness—Overall effectiveness for your practice	1	2	3	4	5	(17)
Total			____			(18)

Table 9-4 The Common Cold

The Family Medicine Center

What is it? Today you have a runny nose, sore throat, dry cough, body aches, a tired feeling, and a fever. That's your cold, and it's caused by *virus*. Most colds last 3-7 days, and then slowly get better. We cannot *cure* colds, but we can help you feel better.

What can I do? 1. *Rest*—if you have a fever (over 101°), you should stay home and quiet. If you don't have a fever, you can go out, but take it easy—your body needs a chance to recover.

       2. *Fluids*—drink plenty of your favorite fluids, such as water, pop, juice, fruit drinks or tea. You don't have to eat solid food if you don't want to.

       3. *Vaporizer*—a cool steam machine placed next to your bed will help relieve your stuffy head and chest.

       4. *Medicines*—

           *Aspirin or Tylenol (acetaminophen) will help keep your fever down (see fever sheet). Take _____ every _____ hrs.

           *Cold medicines may help some symptoms.

           We suggest:

           _____ — _____ every _____ hrs. for

           _____.

           *Antibiotics—*most often they will not help*—a virus does not respond to them.

Call us if: 1. Your fever cannot be brought down below 101° in 3 or 4 hours, or if the fever lasts more than 2 days.

       2. You have more trouble breathing, or what you cough up is yellow or green.

       3. You (or your child) look very sleepy or floppy; or cannot keep fluids down.

       4. Your chief symptom is ear or throat pain.

---

(3) Using the five criteria (i.e., practicality/implementation, relevance/acceptability, content, format, and effectiveness/evaluation), write a patient education handout for use in your training program or private practice.

(4) Using the evaluation form presented in the chapter, assess patient education materials currently used in your office. Also use this form to evaluate commercially prepared materials.

References

Barsky AJ. Hidden reasons some patients visit doctors. Ann Int Med 1981;94: 492–8.

Brunworth D, Rigden S. Patient education for the family. Hagerstown: Harper & Row, 1979.

Chatham MAH, Knapp BL. Patient education handbook. Bowie: Robert J. Brady Co., 1982.

Doak LG, Doak CC. Patient comprehension profiles: recent findings and strategies. Patient Counselling Health Education 1980;2:101–6.

Gadd AS, Norell SE, Kvarnstrom AC, Strandler U. Different media in patient education: the patient's view. In: Leathar DS, Hastings GB, Davies JK, eds. Health education and the media. Oxford: Pergamon Press, 1981, 369–81.

Griffith HW. Instructions for patients. 2nd ed. Philadelphia: WB Saunders, 1975.

Griffith HW. Drug information for patients. Philadelphia: WB Saunders, 1978.

Griffith HW, Mofenson HC, Greensher J, Greensher A. Information and instructions for pediatric patients. Tuscon: Winter Publ., 1980.

Levie WH. Pictorial research: an overview. Viewpoints 1973;49:37–45.

Maslow AH. A theory of human motivation. Psychological Rev 1943;50:370–96.

McCormick RD, Gilson-Parkevich T. Patient and family education: tools, techniques, and theory. New York: John Wiley & Sons, 1979.

McLaughlin HG. SMOG grading—a new readability formula. J Reading 1969:12.

Morris LA, Halperin JA. Effects of written drug information on patient knowledge and compliance: a literature review. Am J Public Health 1979;69:47–52.

National task force on training family physicians in patient education. Patient education: a handbook for teachers. Kansas City: Society of Teachers of Family Medicine, 1979.

Redman BK. The process of patient teaching in nursing. St. Louis: CV Mosby, 1980.

Schiller C, Schreiber RJ, Belkin M. A study of the effectiveness of advertising frequency in magazines. New York: Time Inc., 1982.

STFM Task Force on Patient Education. Patient education: a curriculum for residents. Kansas City: Society of Teachers of Family Medicine, 1982.

Part V

Common Interest Areas

Chapter **10**

The Editorial Process of *Family Medicine**

Joan S. Carmichael and Lynn P. Carmichael

Introduction

The growth and expansion of the journal *Family Medicine* is essential to the relatively new academic discipline of family medicine. While family practice, the clinical arm of family medicine, is well represented by publications aimed toward practicing physicians, *Family Medicine* is the only journal specifically directed toward family medicine educators and scholars. The content is intended for academic physicians and behavioral and social scientists, nurses, social workers, researchers, members of the clergy, and other professionals actively involved in the discipline.

Since *Family Medicine* is the official publication of the Society of Teachers of Family Medicine (STFM) and serves as its voice in matters related to family medicine education, research, and understanding, members should be aware of its editorial procedures and publishing policies. This chapter briefly describes the background, evolution and structure of the journal. The primary purpose of the chapter is to provide an understanding of the journal's current editorial process and to offer suggestions to potential authors and reviewers.

---

*The editorial process described in the following chapter is representative of most peer-review medical journals; in many ways, it presents an ideal to which other publications should aspire. Ed.

Background and Evolution

One of the early objectives of the new multidisciplinary STFM, established in 1967, was to provide a forum to assist in the definition of the discipline and to serve as a medium for exchange of ideas, new methodologies, and educational experiences. During those early years, a tabloid, *Family Practice Times*, later named *Family Medicine Times* (FMT), initially edited by Silas Grant, served as that medium. In 1969, the tabloid was replaced by the *FMT Newsletter* which the STFM retained for the next 10 years.

While the Needs Assessment Survey of the STFM's membership in 1977 clearly indicated the perceived need for a more formal news publication and articulated the need for a refereed journal, such a journal was beyond the financial capability of the Society. In response to the members' needs, however, *Family Medicine Teacher* edited by Lynn Carmichael M.D., replaced the *Newsletter* in January 1979, and served as a bridge to the present more academic journal, *Family Medicine*.

Structure of the Journal

The Society of Teachers of Family Medicine owns and publishes *Family Medicine*. In February 1982, the STFM Board of Directors adopted a policy statement which outlined the organizational responsibilities and authority of the Board, Editor, Communications Committee, Managing Publisher, and the STFM Executive Director in matters regarding the journal. Later that year, the Board appointed 12 members to the Editorial Review Board. In addition, members of both the Communications Committee and the Editorial Review Board serve as manuscript reviewers. All members of STFM receive a subscription to *Family Medicine*. Other subscribers pay a subscription fee determined by the Board and group subscriptions are available.

The Editorial Process

On receipt in the editorial office, all contributions are scanned for appropriateness and suitability for potential publishing in an academic journal. Manuscripts considered by the Editor to be inappropriate to enter the review process are returned to the author with a letter stating the reasons for rejecting the article and, if feasible, inviting the author to resubmit the paper following revisions. Reasons for returning the contribution include excessive length, content more appropriate for a clinical or other specialty journal, lack of proper documentation, incomprehensibility, or such patent scientific flaws that the reason for rejection is obvious. If the manuscript is considered suitable to enter the review process, the Editor selects the reviewers and the author is informed that the paper is under anonymous review. The authors' names, institutions, and other identification are deleted from the manuscript before review.

Manuscripts are sent to the reviewers with a letter asking them to review the paper for its interest, applicability, and importance to academic family medicine. They are asked critically to assess the design, sample selection, methodology, and analysis of research articles. Further, they are requested to complete and return an enclosed evaluation form within 1 month. The evaluation form asks for reviewers' recommendations. Authors are supplied with copies of the reviewers' recommendations along with a letter from the Editor accepting or rejecting their manuscript and editorial comments and suggestions regarding the article. Often, a paper is accepted pending revisions or the reviewers may recommend that a rejected paper be revised and resubmitted for publishing consideration. In this case, the revised paper is reviewed by the same reviewers. Should the reviewers disagree or neglect to return their critique following a second letter or telephone call, the Editor makes the decision regarding publication.

When the author returns the accepted and revised paper, the paper is edited for publication. If the editing is substantial, a copy is returned to the author for approval. When the fate of a manuscript has been decided, the reviewers receive a "thank you" letter as well as a copy of the letter sent to the author (minus identification) and a copy of the other reviewers' recommendations.

The length of time a manuscript may spend in the editorial process depends on a number of factors such as how quickly the reviewers respond, how long it takes the author to revise the manuscript, and the number of manuscripts waiting to be published. Some papers require two or three revisions, a process that, of course, extends the time until publication.

Suggestions for Authors

Organization/Form

The "Information-for-Authors" column in the journal cautions authors not to submit manuscripts that have been submitted or published elsewhere (Huth, 1981). This policy has recently been stated in the International Committee of Medical Journal Editors' (1982), *Uniform Requirements for Manuscripts Submitted to Biomedical Journals*, which forms the basis for information-for-authors pages in more than 150 journals. If authors prepare manuscripts according to the requirements specified in this document, their papers will not be returned for changes in format. The *Uniform Requirements* include information regarding typing instructions, title page, abstract, text, references, tables, illustrations, and abbreviations for frequently cited journals and units of measurement. This document will prove useful to anyone contemplating submitting material to a biomedical journal. While the uniform requirements are invaluable as a guide for the overall form for manuscripts, authors must carefully consult the "Information-for-Authors" column in the journal for specific requirements unique to *Family Medicine*. For example, the journal requires the original and one copy of all submitted contributions.

Style

Manuscripts are more likely to be accepted for publication if the writing is simple, concise, and presented in a logical, clear style (Ableson, 1981; DeBakey, 1976; Lundberg, 1982). Crichton (1975) identified 10 recurring faults in random journal articles from three different issues of the *New England Journal of Medicine*. The faults were: poor flow of ideas, verbage, redundancy, repetition, wrong word, poor syntax, excessive abstraction, unnecessary complexity, excessive compression, and unnecessary qualification. Most of these faults may be found in the contributions to *Family Medicine* as well. Historically, researchers and scientific writers wrote in the third person, passive voice. According to Bem (1981), it is now permissible to use the first person voice, and O'Connor (1979) prefers the active to the passive voice when appropriate. Past tenses should be used when reporting previous research of others and present tense for results currently in front of the reader. Today's authors are expected to avoid language that reinforces sexism (see APA, 1975 Reference for a useful set of guidelines on nonsexist language). Accuracy, brevity, and clarity are characteristics most editors (and reviewers) cherish (Bjork, 1981).

Content

The "Information-for-Authors" statement in each issue of *Family Medicine* encourages readers to submit material for publishing consideration. As noted, scholarly papers germane to the broad field of family medicine are invited. These may include current developments in teaching, education, and position statements, as well as pertinent studies, investigations, and evaluations. Submitted material generally falls into one of four categories—Original Contributions, Special Articles, Brief Reports (a recent addition) and Transactions, the Letters to the Editor section; papers in the first three categories are reviewed anonymously by STFM members, while Transaction items are edited, but not refereed.

Original Contributions

These manuscripts should be clear, succinct, and follow the standardized format used for research articles. This format includes the Abstract, Introduction, Method, Results, Discussion, and References sections (Gelbach, 1982). Bem (1981) suggested that this report is usually written in the "shape" of an hourglass. It begins with broad general statements, progressively narrows down to specifics, and then broadens out again to more general conclusions. Original contributions are refereed by three peers: (1) a member of the Editorial Review Board, (2) a Society member with expertise in the topic and (3) an STFM member chosen from the general membership in order to acquaint members with the reviewing procedures and to provide an equal opportunity for all members to participate as referees.

Special Articles

Manuscripts in this category should be in scholarly form with an abstract, review of the literature, references, and proper documentation. Special articles are refereed anonymously by two Communications Committee members.

Brief Reports

This section includes position statements, committee reports, curriculum descriptions, and other pertinent items. Brief reports are limited to 1,000 words and are refereed by reviewers selected by the editor.

Transactions

Letters to the Editor are accepted for publication without review, provided the editing required is minor and the content relevant. They are limited to around 500 words and are frequently opinion pieces written in response to an article previously published in *Family Medicine*.

Suggestions for Reviewers

Reviewers or referees play a major role in the *Family Medicine* editorial process since their recommendations usually determine whether a manuscript is rejected or accepted for publication. As noted, reviewers are members of the Communications Committee, Editorial Review Board or are randomly selected Society members. Most reviewers give a great deal of time and thought to their critiques as shown by the reviews received in the Editorial Office. Many referees add extra pages of specific suggestions to the evaluation form; other reviewers write comments and questions in the margins of the manuscript; some attach pertinent reprints to their recommendations.

Most authors invest innumerable hours in writing and revising their manuscripts before submitting them for publishing consideration; referees should review papers with open and impartial attitudes (Lock, 1982; Smith, 1982). The manuscript should be considered a privileged document, and reviewers are expected to keep its content confidential. This means the paper must not be photocopied or discussed with colleagues. Reviewers' recommendations should always be written tactfully.

If a reviewer knows that the review will not be completed in the specified 1 month's time, the manuscript should be returned to the editorial office so another referee may be selected. The reviewer should pay attention to the style, syntax, and grammar of the paper. Questions reviewers should consider include: Does the manuscript conform to the Uniform Requirements? Is the content relevant to *Family Medicine*? Does the title and abstract reflect the content of the paper? Are the references adequate and recent?

In a research study, reviewers should ask: Are the problem and the hypothesis clearly stated and is the study designed properly? Are the population and sample appropriate and are the study and control groups comparable? Are data collection and analysis appropriate and are the statistical procedures sound? Do data support the conclusions and are the results generalizable? Finally, are limitations of the study stated?

Although blind peer review may be an arduous task at times, both authors and reviewers benefit from the process. Since the review is anonymous, the manuscript stands on its own merit rather than on the author's reputation or institution. The paper receives an honest and impartial appraisal by two or three of the author's peers as well as editorial comments. These suggestions may help authors in writing their next paper, as well as improving the manuscript under review. *Family Medicine* is unique in that reviewers and authors are provided with copies of all reviewers' critiques and editorial observations. This kind of interchange may help reviewers in sharpening their own writing skills. Reviewers say they receive satisfaction from this kind of feedback. They also report satisfaction when the manuscript they so diligently reviewed is published.

Summary

The chapter briefly describes the background, evolution, and structure of *Family Medicine,* the official publication of STFM. The purpose of the chapter is to explain the journal's editorial process and to provide suggestions for reviewers and authors.

Just as family medicine is continuing to define itself, *Family Medicine* is growing and changing. The quantity of contributions is increasing and the quality of the manuscripts is steadily improving. The editorial office encourages contributions from published and unpublished authors. Ideas and suggestions regarding reviewing procedures are welcome.

References

Ableson PA. Support of scientific journals (Editorial). Science 1981;214.

Anonymous. The craft of shortening. Lancet 1970;2:1077–8.

Anonymous. What kind of journal? (Editorial). J Roy Coll Gen Pract 1980;30:707–11.

APA Task Force on Issues of Sexual Bias in Graduate Education. Guidelines for non-sexist use of language. American Psychologist 1975;30:682–4.

APA Publication Manual Task Force. Publication manual change sheet 2.1977. Washington DC: American Psychological Association.

Bem D. Writing the research report. In: Selltiz C, Wrightsman L, Cook S, eds. Research methods in social relations. New York: Holt, Rinehart and Winston, 1981:342–64.

Bjork RE. The careful writer and the sound of words. J Comm Health 1981;6:275–81.

Crichton M. Medical obfuscation: structure and function. N Engl J Med 1975; 293:1257–9.

DeBakey L. The scientific journal: editorial policies and practices. St. Louis: CV Mosby Co, 1976.

Gehlbach SH. Interpreting the medical literature. Lexington, Mass.: DC Health and Co, 1982.

Huth EJ. The ethics of medical publishing: prior publication and full disclosure by authors (editorial). Ann Int Med 1981;94:401–2.

International Committee of Medical Journal Editors. Uniform requirements for manuscripts submitted to biomedical journals. Ann Intern Med 1982;96:766–70.

Lock S. Peer review weighed in the balance. Br Med J 1982;285:1124–6.

Lundberg GD. Goals for the journal (Editorial). J Am Med Assoc 1982;248:553.

O'Conner M, ed. The scientist as editor. New York: John Wiley, 1979.

Smith R. Steaming up windows and refereeing medical papers. Br Med J 1982;285:1259–61.

Chapter 11

Selected Publishing Sources in Family Medicine

Jane Barclay Mandel

A variety of publishing sources exists for the person interested in reaching an audience in family medicine or family practice. These include journals on clinical practice emphasizing treatment of specific cases and new methods of patient care, medical education emphasizing undergraduate didactic teaching and research on educational methodology, as well as teaching approaches and evaluation in clinical settings. Other journals emphasize various aspects of research as it bears upon family medicine. This may be in the area of epidemiology, delivery of services, clinical trials, or the interaction of psychological and physical approaches (behavioral medicine). Many journals include articles of opinion and theory on medical economics, social issues that affect health care and medicolegal issues, and review articles on the history and philosophy of medicine and medical ethics. Most journals publish brief commentary or reactions to articles as letters to the editor. A few also solicit poetry or short prose pieces.

The journals relevant to family practice are drawn from a wide-ranging number of disciplines including, of course, family medicine and the related specialties of pediatrics, obstetrics, and gynecology, medicine, psychology, and psychiatry, as well as sociology, health care delivery, public health, and epidemiology.

Many of these journals are new, and as a result, they are not yet included in the *Index Medicus* system. Identifying publication sources relevant to family medicine, then, can be difficult and may be limited to the journals to which one already subscribes. The Family Medicine Literature Index (FAMLI) has attempted to bridge this gap by indexing a group of journals relevant to primary care family medicine. When looking for a publishing source, the FAMLI can be an excellent place to begin. The Subject Index will provide citations and journal sources on a particular topic.

The type of communication desired by an author may also influence the journal sought. Brief communications, case studies, and reports of clinical techniques may be reported as special communication or transaction articles. Research articles following the format outlined in other chapters in this book are appropriately sent to some journals while other publications focus on clinical applications and practical therapeutics. Thorough review articles are also appropriate submissions. Theoretical articles which may include a literature review or may simply be a fresh discussion of a topical problem are also sought. Many journals accept book or media reviews, and all publish letters to the editor.

The listings below summarize a grouping of journals relevant to family medicine. The listings provide the frequency of publication, categories of articles accepted by each journal, and information about the format in which written material should be submitted. Many of these journals use the Uniform Requirements for Manuscripts Submitted to Biomedical Journals (see Appendix). Journals choose their major articles by peer review often using members of their editorial board. Unless otherwise indicated, the journals below use the peer review process. Acceptance of letters to the editor, book reviews, and brief commentary are generally at the discretion of the editor. This listing should provide a helpful guide for the author in search of publication.

AMERICAN FAMILY PHYSICIAN
American Academy of Family Physicians
1740 West 92nd Street
Kansas City, Missouri 64114

Issued monthly at $40.00 per year. Free to AAFP members.
Publishes original articles which focus on practical aspects of medical science and also current concepts and developments in other specialties, including basic science reviews. Does not publish detailed reports of experimental studies.
Uses Uniform Requirements for Manuscripts Submitted to Biomedical Journals.
Editorial advisory board.

ANNALS OF INTERNAL MEDICINE
American College of Physicians
4200 Pine Street

Philadelphia, Pennsylvania 19104
(215) 243-1200   (800) 523-1546

Issued monthly at $45.00 per year.
Publishes articles or short papers (1,500 words) on etiology, pathology, epidemiology, diagnosis, or treatment of disease; brief reports (750 words) on clinical trials, studies, or cases; papers on medical education, social and political issues related to medicine, review articles, clinical applications; book and journal reviews, prose and poetry (900 words/80 lines), and letters to the editor (400 words).
Uses the Uniform Requirements for Manuscripts Submitted to Biomedical Journals.
Editors and consultants provide review.

ARCHIVES OF INTERNAL MEDICINE
American Medical Association
535 North Dearborn Street
Chicago, Illinois 60610

Issued monthly, included in AMA membership dues; nonmembers, $30.00 per year.
Publishes editorial articles, original investigations, clinical management, review articles, and book reviews. Single case reports are not solicited.
Uses the Uniform Requirements for Manuscripts Submitted to Biomedical Journals and the AMA Manuscript Manual for Authors and Editors.
Editorial board.

CANADIAN MEDICAL ASSOCIATION JOURNAL
Canadian Medical Association
P.O. Box 8650
Ottawa, Ontario K1G 0G8

Issued twice monthly to Canadian Medical Association members.
Individual U.S. subscription rate, $69.00 per year.
Publishes clinical and scientific aspects of medicine, medical education, medical economics, medicolegal affairs, health care delivery, history of medicine. Typical article length, 3,000 word maximum; brief communication, 1,000 words or less; letters to the editor, 500 words or less.
Uses the Uniform Requirements for Manuscripts Submitted to Biomedical Journals; published in English and French.
Editorial board.

CONTINUING EDUCATION FOR THE FAMILY PHYSICIAN
Le Jacq Publishing, Inc.
53 Park Place
New York, New York 10007

Manuscripts should be sent to:
G. Gayle Stephens, M.D.
Department of Family Practice
UAB Medical Center
University Station
Birmingham, Alabama 35294

Issued monthly at $40.00 per year.
Publishes articles (1500–5000 words) which are invited from family physicians, other specialists and clinics on clinical topics of practical value; book reviews; letters (600 word maximum).
Proper format can be found in the current issue.

EMERGENCY MEDICINE
Fischer Medical Publications, Inc.
280 Madison Avenue
New York, New York 10016
(212) 889-4530

Issued semimonthly at $25.00–$32.50, U.S. individual rate.
Publishes articles pertaining to emergency medicine, diagnosis, treatment, and research; letters to the editor.
Uses the Uniform Requirements for Manuscripts Submitted to Biomedical Journals.
Editorial advisory board.

EVALUATION AND THE HEALTH PROFESSIONS
Sage Publications, Inc.
275 South Beverly Drive
Beverly Hills, California 90212

Issued quarterly at $22.00 per year, U.S. individual rate.
Publishes results of evaluation studies, instructional innovations, progress reports, and updates. Solicits from all health professionals. Maximum length of articles, 30 double-spaced pages.
Uses the American Statistical, Psychological, and Sociological Association style sheets, available from the publisher.
Editorial board.

FAMILY MEDICINE
Society of Teachers of Family Medicine
1740 West 92nd Street
Kansas City, Missouri 64114
(816) 333-9700

Issued six times a year (January, March, May, July, September, and November) to STFM members. Nonmembers, $30.00 per year.
Publishes articles of interest to family medicine including research and education; book and media reviews. Article length, 3000 words; transactions, 500 words.
Uses the Uniform Requirements for Manuscripts Submitted to Biomedical Journals.
Editorial board.

FAMILY PRACTICE RECERTIFICATION
Medical Recertification Association
2 Park Avenue
New York, New York 10016
(212) 689-3777

Issued monthly at $30.00, U.S. individual rate.
Publishes updated information including assessment and problem-solving, patient management and follow-up techniques for the practicing family physician (3,000 words).
Proper format can be found in the current issue.
Editorial board.

FAMILY PRACTICE RESEARCH JOURNAL
(Co-sponsored by Michigan Academy of Family Physicians and The Family Health Research, Education, and Service Institute)
Human Sciences Press
72 Fifth Avenue
New York, New York 10011
(212) 243-6000

Issued quarterly at $28.00 per year.
Publishes articles on research in family medicine and medical education with a research/evaluation component. Papers can be experimental, historical, basic research, clinical research, or case studies. The journal will assist authors in paper preparation through review commentary.
Proper format can be found in the current issue.
Editorial board.

HEALTH PSYCHOLOGY
Journal of the Division of Health Psychology, American Psychological Association
Lawrence Erlbaum Associates, Ind.
365 Broadway, Suite 102
Hillsdale, New Jersey 07642

Issued quarterly at $19.50 per year.

Publishes reports of empirical research on aspects of the health system, evaluations of psychological interventions, health policy issue analysis from a psychological standpoint; reviews of the literature and methodological papers; book reviews.

Uses the Publication Manual of the American Psychologial Association, 2nd Edition.

Editorial board.

HOSPITAL AND COMMUNITY PSYCHIATRY
American Psychiatric Association
1700 18th Street NW
Washington, D.C. 20009

Issued monthly at $27.00, U.S. individual rate.

Publishes a broad range of articles including liaison psychiatry, clinical management, community mental health, health policy, and legal aspects (3,000 words); brief reports (1,200 words); Open Forum, a section of commentary and opinion (300–800 words); letters to the editor (500 words); book reviews.

Proper format can be found in the current issue.

Editorial board.

JOURNAL OF THE AMERICAN GERIATRIC SOCIETY
American Geriatrics Society
W. B. Saunders Company
West Washington Square
Philadelphia, Pennsylvania 19105

Issued monthly at $50.00 per year.

Publishes original articles (2,000–4,000 words) on clinical or research subjects, clinical reports (500–1,400 words), review articles (3,000–10,000 words), and letters (250–500 words); book reviews.

Proper format can be found in the current issue.

Editorial board.

JAMA
American Medical Association
535 Dearborn Street
Chicago, Illinois 60610
(312) 751-6000

Issued four times per month; subscription rate included in AMA annual dues; nonmembers, $52.00 per year.

Publishes major articles, brief reports (1,500–1,800 words), clinical notes (600–700 words); letters to the editor.
Uses the Uniform Requirements for Manuscripts Submitted to Biomedical Journals and the AMA Manuscript Manual for Authors and Editors.
Editorial board.

THE JOURNAL OF FAMILY PRACTICE
Appleton–Century–Crofts, A Division of Prentice–Hall, Inc.
25 Van Zant Street
East Norwalk, Connecticut 06855
(203) 838-4400

Issued monthly at $40.00 per year, U.S. individual rate.
Publishes original articles, feature articles, letters to the editor, position papers; topics include clinical care, health care delivery, education, and research which advance and define the discipline of family medicine; book reviews.
Proper format can be found in the current issue.
Editorial board and editorial advisory board.

JOURNAL OF HUMAN STRESS
Helen Dwight Reid Educational Foundation
4000 Albemarle Street, N.W.
Washington, D.C. 20016

Issued quarterly at $33.00 per year.
Publishes articles which investigate environmental and emotional influences on behavior and health, and the course of physical disorders in humans; articles (15 pages maximum); letters to the editor.
Uses the *Index Medicus* reference style; proper format can be found in the current issue.
Editorial board.

JOURNAL OF MEDICAL EDUCATION
Association of American Medical Colleges
One Dupont Circle, N.W.
Washington, D.C. 20036
(202) 828-0640

Issued monthy at $33.00 per year, U.S. individual rate.
Publishes major articles (15 double-spaced pages), communications (four pages), briefs (250 words), letters to the editor (2 pages); book reviews.
Proper format can be found in the current issue.
Editorial board.

THE JOURNAL OF PEDIATRICS
The C. V. Mosby Company
11830 Westline Industrial Drive
St. Louis, Missouri 63141
(217) 789-4204

Issued monthly at $40.50 per year, U.S. individual rate.
Publishes original research, clinical observations and reviews of pediatric
subjects and related fields; letters to the editor; book reviews. No lengths
given.
Uses the *Index Medicus* style for references. Proper format can be found in
the current issue.
Editorial board.

JOURNAL OF THE ROYAL COLLEGE OF GENERAL PRACTITIONERS
8 Queen Street
Edinburgh EH2 1JE, Scotland
(Published by Update Publications Ltd., 33/44 Alfred Place, London WCIE
7DP). (Manuscripts are sent to Edinburgh.)

Issued monthly at $100 per year, U.S. postfree rate.
Subscription price includes Reports from General Practice and Journal
Supplements.
Publishes original articles, editorials, case studies, surveys, letters to the
editor.
Proper format can be found in the current issue in "editorial notice."
Editorial board.

LANCET
Little, Brown, and Company
24 Beacon Street
Boston, Massachusetts 02106

Issued weekly at $65.00 per year.
Publishes original articles, preliminary communications (1,500 words),
methods and devices (750 words), letters to the editor (500 words), book
reviews, articles on special topics (e.g., occupational health, toxicology,
nutrition, public health).
Uses the Uniform Requirements for Manuscripts Submitted to Biomedical
Journals.
Articles reviewed by the London editorial office.

MEDICAL CARE
J. B. Lippincott Company
East Washington Square

Philadelphia, Pennsylvania 19105
(Offical publication of the Medical Care Section of the American Public
Health Association)

Issued monthly at $48.00 per year, U.S. individual rate.
Publishes articles in the broad field of medical care to encourage progress
in the research, planning, organization, financing, provision, and evalua-
tion of health services.
Uses of Uniform Requirements for Manuscripts Submitted to Biomedical
Journals.
Editorial board.

MEDICAL EDUCATION
Blackwell Scientific Publications, Ltd.
9 Forrest Road
Edinburgh EH1 2QH, Scotland

Issued bimonthly to members of the Association for the Study of Medical
Education; $120 per year, U.S. individual rate, via air.
Publishes exchanges of information on undergraduate, postgraduate, and
continuing medical education.
Proper format can be found in the current issue. References use the
Harvard system, i.e., name followed by date in parentheses.

MEDICAL TIMES
Romain Pierson Publishers, Inc.
80 Shore Road
Port Washington, New York 11050
(516) 883-6350

Issued monthly at $35.00 per year, U.S. individual rate.
Publishes Professorial Pearls: brief clinical examples or explanations used
in teaching clinical family medicine (10–500 words maximum). Does not
actively solicit, but does accept original clinical articles; Anecdotal
Antidotes: brief amusing real-life happenings related to clinical medicine,
previously unpublished.
Write to editor for style guide.
Editorial board.

NEW ENGLAND JOURNAL OF MEDICINE
10 Shattuck Street
Boston, Massachusetts 02115

Issued weekly at $55.00 per year.
Publishes original articles, brief reports, correspondence, and book

reviews. No lengths specified.

Uses the Uniform Requirements for Manuscripts Submitted to Biomedical Journals and the Council of Biology Editors Style Manual, 4th Edition, Arlington, Virginia, American Institute of Biological Sciences, 1978. Authors may suggest reviewers.

PATIENT CARE: The Practical Journal for Primary Care Physicians
Patient Care Communications, Inc.
16 Thorndal Circle
P.O. Box 1245
Darien, Connecticut 06820
(203) 655-8951

Issued on the 15th and 30th monthly except July, August, and December, when published on the 15th; $42.00 per year.

Publishes invited articles and round tables only; letters to the editor; reviewer comments on major articles.

Contact editor for proper format.

Board of Editors, Special Consultants, and Advisory Board.

PATIENT COUNSELLING AND HEALTH EDUCATION
Exerpta Medica
P.O. Box 3085
Princeton, New Jersey 08540
(609) 896-9450

Issued quarterly at $18.50 per year.

Publishes original articles in patient education, counselling, health risk reduction programs including descriptive, evaluation, and research approaches.

Proper format can be found in current issue.

Editorial Board.

PEDIATRICS
American Academy of Pediatrics
P.O. Box 1034
Evanston, Illinois 60204

Issued monthly at $42.00 per year.

Publishes major articles, review articles, clinical notes, and letters to the editor.

Uses the Uniform Requirements for Manuscripts Submitted to Biomedical Journals and the AMA Manuscript Manual for Authors and Editors.

Editorial board.

POSTGRADUATE MEDICINE: The Journal of Applied Medicine for the Primary
 Care Physician
McGraw Hill
4530 West 77th Street
Minneapolis, Minnesota 55435
(612) 835-3222

Issued monthly at $38.00 per year.
Publishes original papers in all medical fields, presented to be of interest to
the primary care physician (2,000 words); book reviews.
Uses the Uniform Requirements for Manuscripts Submitted to Biomedical
Journals.
Editorial board.

PREVENTIVE MEDICINE
American Health Foundation, published by Academic Press
320 East 43rd Street
New York, New York 10017

Issued bimonthly at $110.00 per year.
Publishes original manuscripts dealing with applied research on preven-
tion, emphasizing cancer, stroke, heart disease, and preventable causes of
death (20 pages maximum).
Proper format can be found in the current issue.
Editorial board.

PSYCHOSOMATIC MEDICINE
American Psychosomatic Society
265 Nassau Road
Roosevelt, New York 11575

Issued bimonthly at $54.00 per year.
Publishes original articles on research, review articles, short inputs, book
reviews.
Proper format can be found in the Annual May-June issue.
Editorial board.

PSYCHOSOMATICS, Journal of the Academy of Psychosomatic Medicine
Cligott Publishing Company
500 West Putnam Street
Greenwich, Connecticut 06830
(203) 661-0600

Issued monthly at $20.00 per year.
Publishes original articles on the interrelationship of psychiatry and

medical practice (3,000 words), psychosomatic case reports (1,200 words), brief letters to the editor.

Uses AMA Manuscript Manual for Authors and Editors.

Consulting and advisory editors; peer review.

References

A compilation of journal instructions to authors. Bethesda: National Cancer Institute, 1979.

AMA manuscript manual for authors & editors, 7th ed. Los Altos: Lange Medical Publications, 1981.

Directory of publishing opportunities in journals and periodicals, 4th ed. Chicago: Marquis Academic Media, 1979.

Family medicine literature index, v. 1—, WONCA, March 1980.

Meiss HR, Jaeger DA, eds. Information to authors 1980–81. Baltimore/Munich: Urban & Schwarzenberg, 1980.

Roberts MC, Lyman RC, Breiner J, Royal GP. Publishing child-oriented articles in psychology:: A compendium of publication outlets. Washington, D.C.: University Press of America, Inc., 1982.

Uniform requirements for manuscripts submitted to biomedical journals. Ann Intern Med 1982;96(1):766–71.

Uniform requirements for manuscripts submitted to biomedical journals. Brit Med J 1982, 284:1766–70.

Chapter 12

A Short, Annotated Bibliography for Authors of Medical, Scientific, and Other Scholarly Articles

Thomas E. Crowder

Introduction

During the compilation of this bibliography, I have read—or examined with a great degree of care—over 100 books and articles on scientific writing. The selections that follow are, in my opinion, among the most practical ones I have found. They were chosen for their potential usefulness to authors of clinical articles as well as to those who would write for journals like *Family Medicine*, which are more academically and theoretically oriented. The selections reflect my biases and ideas of what is useful. Inevitably, many other valuable and informative books and articles have been omitted; this is intended to be no judgment on their merits but rather it is the result of space constraints.

I have restricted entries mainly to books, because bibliographical information about articles in journals is readily available through *Index Medicus* and other bibliographic control devices.

I was both heartened and discouraged while I was doing the work of compiling the bibliography. I was heartened because by far the greater portion of the materials I read was to be found in the Calder Memorial Library of the University of Miami School of Medicine; I was discouraged because none of them seems to have been checked out.

With sincere hopes that this bibliography will be helpful and widely used, I would like to remind authors and would-be authors that one of the most important articles on scientific writing for authors to read is the

196 T. E. Crowder

"Information to Authors" section of the journal to which they intend to submit a manuscript.

● AMERICAN PSYCHOLOGICAL ASSOCIATION. APA PUBLICATION MANUAL TASK FORCE. GUIDELINES FOR NONSEXIST LANGUAGE IN APA JOURNALS (PUBLICATION MANUAL CHANGE SHEET 2, JUNE 1977). AMERICAN PSYCHOLOGIST, JUNE 1977, P. 487–494.

This is one to the standards enjoined upon authors of articles submitted to *Family Medicine*. It offers general principles for authors to consider, and suggests ways to avoid sexist language. Its general purpose is to help writers of journal articles develop a style devoid of sexist and stereotypical constructions, and to help authors toward accurate, unbiased communication. It also is a minicourse in sensitivity to some of the cultural issues embedded in our habitual use of language. Further, the paper demonstrates that nonsexist language need not be infelicitous.

● BARCLAY, W. R., SOUTHGATE, M. T., AND MAYO, R. W., COMPS. MANUAL FOR AUTHORS AND EDITORS: EDITORIAL STYLE AND MANUSCRIPT PREPARATION. COMPILED FOR THE AMERICAN MEDICAL ASSOCIATION. LOS ALTOS, CALIF.: LANGE MEDICAL PUBLICATIONS, 1980.

This is the manual used as a standard by the editors of *Family Medicine*. It is most useful for deciding matters of style, such as punctuation, symbols and abbreviations, mathematical and statistical usages, and units of measure, among other similar technical questions. Folks interested in matters dealing with manuscript preparation, planning a paper, and the actual process of getting a paper published will find more help in books such as those by R. A. Day and Lester S. King (annotated elsewhere in this bibliography). Some of the guidelines in this manual are not consistent with other manuals, such as that of the *Council of Biology Editors Style Manual*; however, because the AMA does endorse many widely accepted canons of style, the *Manual* is a useful reference tool, especially for contributors to *Family Medicine*.

● CBE STYLE MANUAL COMMITTEE. COUNCIL OF BIOLOGY EDITORS STYLE MANUAL: A GUIDE FOR AUTHORS, EDITORS, AND PUBLISHERS IN THE BIOLOGICAL SCIENCES. 4TH ED. ARLINGTON: COUNCIL OF BIOLOGY EDITORS, 1978.

This is a manual that has been prepared for authors and editors as well as others who work in the production of literature in the biomedical and biological sciences. It deals with the writing, editing, and publishing of the varied forms of this kind of publication: journal articles, research reports, theses and dissertations, and books, as well as with the various types of articles that may be included in journals.

The manual is concerned primarily with the writing of articles for publication in journals; however, its approach is broad and much of its content is relevant to the writing of other kinds of materials. Chapters cover such topics as getting manuscripts into print, proof correction, the mechanics of indexing, and style in special fields of the biological sciences. There is a helpful "Annotated Bibliography" of other manuals for further reference. Some of the recommendations in the *Manual* differ from those in the AMA style manual.

This manual is extremely helpful with guidance in planning and with the process of writing a paper. It is highly recommended for serious writers of scientific articles or books.

● DAY, ROBERT A. HOW TO WRITE AND PUBLISH A SCIENTIFIC PAPER. PHILADELPHIA: ISI PRESS, 1979.

This is an unabashed "how-to" book, one to which the author brings experience as a teacher of scientific writing, 25 years as a managing editor, and activity in the Council of Biology Editors. The advice given is concrete and practical, covering such subjects as the preparation of effective illustrations; the design of informative tables; ethics, rights, and permissions; and the writing of conference reports, review papers, and theses. Useful chapters on common errors in English and appendices dealing with abbreviations and common errors in style round out the volume. The style is easy to read and witty, and the book can be read straight through as a textbook. A detailed index makes referring to specific topics easy. This book is highly recommended as a practical guide.

Note: The second edition (1983) of this book has recently been issued, but was not available for examination prior to compilation of this bibliography.

● DIRCKX, JOHN H., M.D. DX + RX: A PHYSICIAN'S GUIDE TO MEDICAL WRITING. BOSTON: G.K. HALL & CO., 1977.

Beginning with a chapter entitled, "The Anatomy of Language," Dirckx covers the course of preparing a manuscript for publication, closing the book with "Faults of Concept and Style." Between these poles lie sections on the organization of a paper, clarity, readability, and a useful chapter on the "pathology of language," covering such subjects as argot, inexactness, verbal equivocation, and redundancy.

The book was conceived as a guide for "those who write but seldom for publication"; however, as the writer hoped it would be, the volume is useful for the more sophisticated and experienced writer who needs a quick review of systems from time to time.

Dirckx's style is clear and the book is easy, even entertaining, to read—especially the chapter on "Faults of Syntax" and the last chapter. When this book was written, Dirckx was Medical Director, Student Health Center, University of Dayton in Ohio.

● FOLLET, W. MODERN AMERICAN USAGE, ED. AND COMP. BY BARZUN, J., ET AL. NEW YORK: HILL AND WANG, 1966.

Though this book is neither as comprehensive nor as informative or lively as Fowler's, it is still valuable to the writer.

Follett is sensitive to the nuances of English as it is spoken and written by Americans, and was himself a teacher, writer, and editor of some accomplishment. Of particular interest are his short introductory essays, "On Usage, Purism, and Pedantry," "On the Need of an Orderly Mind," and "On the Need of Some Grammar." His treatment of the abominable adverbial absolute "hopefully" is one that I hope everyone will read and, I hope, take to heart.

The book is readable and its logical arrangement makes it easy to use. Appendices deal with discussions of usages, such as those governing *shall* and *will*, *should* and *would*, and the conventions of punctuation.

Follett began working on *Modern American Usage* in 1959. He died in 1963, before his work on this book was finished. It was completed by Jacques Barzun and a group of other distinguished writers and teachers of English.

● FOWLER, H. W. A DICTIONARY OF MODERN ENGLISH USAGE. 2ND ED., REVISED BY SIR ERNEST GOWERS. OXFORD: CLARENDON PRESS, 1965.

Henry Fowler was called by one of his contemporaries "an instinctive grammatical moralizer," a description which Fowler welcomed. Fowler was a craftsman of language and his moralizing resulted from his attempts to realize high standards in English prose.

This is an idiosyncratic book, reflecting the opinions, biases, and prejudices of the author; yet, it is all the more valuable for that. Fowler was a lover of language and, possessing instincts toward perfection, attempted to reach toward the perfections of felicity and clarity in his own writings and to help point the way to these same perfections for other writers.

The dictionary is awkwardly arranged and not easy to use. Fowler's opinions may be—and have been—challenged. Sometimes the language he uses seems unduly circuitous. Still, the book retains its value as a reference work and will repay in pleasure and sensitivity to language anyone who browses about in it. Especially commended as examples of entries which provide enjoyment and the flavor of Fowler's writing are "split infinitive," and "preposition at end," and "if and when." However, it will be fun to look about in the dictionary and find your own favorites.

This book should be owned and read by any serious writer of English, whether the author's efforts be directed toward technical writing or belles lettres.

● KING, L. S. WHY NOT SAY IT CLEARLY: A GUIDE TO SCIENTIFIC WRITING. BOSTON: LITTLE, BROWN AND COMPANY, 1978.

Lester S. King is former Senior Editor and later Contributing Editor to the Journal of the American Medical Association. He is now retired.

This book, distilled from Dr. King's many years as a journal editor and teacher of scientific writing, is an attempt to "induce in the reader the ability to discriminate good writing from bad, to develop a gut reaction against whatever is clumsy and unclear, to identify specific factors that make bad writing bad, and then to effect improvement." This is an ambitious project and one which King has done his best to make successful. All that is needful is the commitment of the reader. Dr. King's audience is specifically writers of medical articles, but his scope is much wider and applies to expository writing of any kind. He includes treatments of such subjects as syntax, dialects, jargon, starting to write, and setting up a course on writing. A detailed index makes the book useful as a quick reference for specific subjects.

● LANE, N. D., AND KRAMMERER, K. L. WRITER'S GUIDE TO MEDICAL JOURNALS. CAMBRIDGE, MASS: BALLINGER PUBLISHING COMPANY, 1975.

This bibliography is similar in content and intention to *Information to Authors, 1980–1981*, but its entries include titles in the allied health professions and some specialty journals which are not primarily clinical in their orientation. In addition, a cross section of major foreign journals, primarily from Western Europe and from English speaking countries, is included; therefore, some titles included here do not appear in *Information to Authors*.

For each entry, the name and address of the person to whom manuscripts should be submitted is indicated, as well as:

(1) Publication lag time.
(2) Percentage of articles accepted for publication from among the total number of articles submitted.
(3) Journal issue or intervals at which instructions to authors usually appear.
(4) Recommended style manuals and sources for standards.
(5) Instructions to authors, and the date of the journal issue from which the instructions were reproduced or known to be in effect. Instructions to authors over 10 pages in length are either reproduced in part, or the source from which the instructions may be obtained is cited.

There is a permuted title index as an aid for those who may not be sure of the title of the journal for which they are searching. Also included is a section including complete bibliographical citation and sources for specific style manuals and standards.

This volume will be updated and expanded as need dictates.

● MEISS, H. R., AND JAEGER, D. A. INFORMATION TO AUTHORS, 1980–1981: EDITORIAL GUIDELINES REPRODUCED FROM 246 MEDICAL JOURNALS. BALTIMORE: URBAN & SCHWAR-ZENBERG, INC., 1980.

Medical journals vary widely in their stylistic differences. This volume includes reproductions of over 240 of the editorial guidelines issued by medical journals and is intended to enable prospective authors "to select potential publishers and prepare acceptable manuscripts in the most efficient manner."

Journals included are clinical in scope, and include publications of the British Medical Association and a number of international journals in which a high percentage of American authorship is represented. Entries are arranged alphabetically by their National Library of Medicine title abbreviation. The authors have also provided a list of journals by subject and a table of journal characteristics. This table includes circulation figures for each journal where these data are obtainable, a feature which is useful for writers whose choice of a journal may be influenced by the size of the potential audience, and an indication of journals indexed in the 1980 *Index Medicus*.

Three useful appendices include a copy of the "Uniform Requirements for Manuscripts" which are adhered to—either in whole or in part—by an increasing number of journals, including *Family Medicine*. "Recommendations of the World Medical Association: Guiding Medical Doctors in Bio-Medical Research Involving Human Subjects," containing the Declaration of Helsinki as revised in The Declaration of Tokyo, sets forth principles which many editors require in the preparation of manuscripts.

Appendix III includes a listing of style manuals and guides most often cited throughout the journal instructions included in the bibliography.

● MCCAFFERY, M. WRITING THAT'S WORTH READING: A PRACTICAL GUIDE FOR WRITERS OF MEDICAL ARTICLES. CANADIAN FAMILY PHYSICIAN, VOL. 26, PP. 429–32 (MAR 1980); PP. 585–7 (APR 1980); PP. 749–51 (MAY 1980); PP. 872–8 (JUNE 1980); PP. 969–72 (JUL 1980); PP. 1064–6 (AUG. 1980).

This is a series of six articles by the editor of *Canadian Family Physician*. It presents a "step by step guide to preparing a manuscript for publication, from index cards to publication." Mrs. McCaffery takes potential authors through these steps with elegance and wit. The articles are easy to read, are succinct, and a reading of them should be of value to the neophyte as well as to the seasoned writer. The series is highly recommended, as much for its inside look at the editorial process as for its practical and down-to-earth advice for authors.

The series concludes with a bibliography of books useful to authors of medical articles. A germane editorial entitled "Superfluous Redundancy" appears in *Can. Fam. Physician* for February 1982 (Vol. 28, pp. 174), and two letters written in reply to the editorial can be found in *Can. Fam. Physician* for May 1982 (Vol. 28: pp. 844–846). These letters are informative and amusing.

● O'CONNOR, M., AND WOODFORD, F. P. WRITING SCIENTIFIC PAPERS IN ENGLISH. NEW YORK: AMERICAN ELSEVIER, 1975.

This is a guide for authors of "any nationality who want to submit papers to journals published in English." Intended for writers whose native language is not English, the book is also useful for those of us who naturally speak American English or who slip easily into the arcane languages of Medicine or Philosophy, and such other "foreign" tongues.

Chapters cover such subjects as planning, preparing and writing the first draft, and carry the reader through the entire process of publication to correcting the proofs. Five appendices are entitled, "Steps in Writing a Paper," "Units of Measure and their Abbreviations," "General Abbreviations and Symbols," "Abbreviations in Biochemistry and Taxonomy," and "Expressions to Avoid." A bibliography of materials on writing, including American, British, and International Standards rounds out this admirable volume. Guidelines given in the work conform in general to the recommendations to authors in the *CBE Style Manual* and are consistent with relevant standards listed in the bibliography. Maeve O'Connor is Senior Editor, Ciba Foundation, London, and she and Woodford have produced a book that can be recommended to both inexperienced writers and veterans of the paper chase.

● ORWELL, G. "POLITICS AND THE ENGLISH LANGUAGE," IN: A COLLECTION OF ESSAYS BY GEORGE ORWELL. NEW YORK: HARCOURT BRACE JOVANOVICH, PUBLISHERS, 1954.

Those who know George Orwell only as the author of *1984* and *Animal Farm* might be astonished to learn that he was one of the most accomplished essayists to write in English in the twentieth century. "Politics and the English Language" deals primarily with the obfuscatory uses of English to which we are all sometimes prone. Orwell was noted for the clarity and vigor of his prose style, and the rules that he lays down here are commonsense ones that were tested in the crucible of the writer's marketplace. Orwell's strictures are designed to produce "language as an instrument for expressing and not for concealing or preventing thought." They deserve attention, for they evolved out of the experience of a writer who succeeded in using words as just this sort of tool and who writes about language as a man who loves and respects it. This essay is short, meaty, and entertaining as well as informative. It is highly recommended. Although the entire essay is a political tract, one need not agree with the politician in order to learn from the writer.

● STRUNK, W., JR. THE ELEMENTS OF STYLE. 3RD ED. REVISED AND EDITED BY E. B. WHITE. NEW YORK: THE MACMILLAN COMPANY, 1979.

This little book, consisting of fewer than one hundred pages, is one which should be in the library—to be read and then read again—of all who would see their words in print. Strunk originally prepared the book as a classbook for an English course at Cornell University, a course in which

White, who later became a writer of note, was a student. *The Elements of Style* has become deservedly famous as a practical guide to a succinct, clear, and vital writing style. The book was originally issued in 1918 and is still in print. That there is currently a paperback edition available, is testimony to its usefulness. The book is, however, probably more useful to the writer of essays, narrative accounts, and such, than it would be to the author of a "purely scientific" exposition. Nevertheless, anyone who aspires to a graceful, brief, and vigorous writing style should have it and read it. It is a classic of its genre.

● UNIVERSITY OF CHICAGO PRESS. A MANUAL OF STYLE, 12TH ED., REV. CHICAGO, UNIVERSITY OF CHICAGO PRESS, 1969.

This edition of a volume which was first issued in 1906 in a considerably more modest form is essentially a new book, although, according to its editors, it is built upon the foundation of earlier versions.

A Manual of Style would be of most value to authors of books; however, its value to writers of articles should not be overlooked. The book treats a truly comprehensive array of ordinary subjects, ranging from punctuation to abbreviations. It also covers more abstruse matters, such as foreign languages in type, standard signs and symbols, preparation of tables, scaling and cropping of artwork, captions and legends, the preparation of an index, and type styles.

The book is intended for use by authors, editors, and copywriters, and is one of the more useful and informative reference works available. It is logically arranged and easy to use.

● WOODFORD, F. P., ED. SCIENTIFIC WRITING FOR GRADUATE STUDENTS: A MANUAL ON THE TEACHING OF SCIENTIFIC WRITING. NEW YORK: ROCKEFELLER UNIVERSITY PRESS, 1968.

A Council of Biology Editors Manual prepared by the CBE Committee on Graduate Training in Scientific Writing.

This volume is addressed to teachers of scientific writing, and results from the awareness of the members of the Council of Biology Editors ... (that) ... many scientists write "badly" and their desire to remedy the hiatus in university curricula that perpetuates this situation. Members of the council have tried to collect in one volume the "widely scattered source materials and references necessary for the preparation of a course (in scientific writing) and to provide a curricular outline from which instructors who may be under pressure of other duties can work with a minimum of preparation."

Chapters 1–10 in the book contain a detailed course in scientific writing, which can be given in about 12 one-hour sessions. Chapters 11–14 deal with "Preparation for Writing the Doctoral Thesis," "Writing a Research Project Proposal," "Oral Presentation of a Scientific Paper," and "Principles and Practices in Searching the Scientific Literature."

The instructions given in the book are practical, down-to-earth and clearly written. Each chapter incorporates suggested readings from appropriate reference materials and presents its matter in a logical, step-by-step fashion. A list of essential text books is given and a brief annotated bibliography of further reading rounds out the volume.

Although the book is directed toward classroom teachers of writing, it could be used as a self-teaching aid for aspiring writers of scientific papers, provided enough discipline were brought to the task; in any case, reading the book would be a worthy endeavor for any writer or teacher of writing.

Appendix I

Table I. Exercises Useful in Writing Skills Workshops

Table IA. Article Organization Exercise

The group should select a topic. Each participant develops a two- or three-part outline with subheadings, as well as a working title and opening sentence.

Topic: _____

Outline: Major heading I.: _____

         Subheadings A. _____

                    B. _____

                    C. _____

      Major heading II.: _____

         Subheadings A. _____

                    B. _____

                    C. _____

      Major heading III.: _____

                    A. _____

                    B. _____

                    C. _____

Table IA *(continued)*

Title: _____

Opening Sentence: _____

_____

_____
_____

Table IB.   Composition Exercise[a]

The group should select a topic and develop an outline of major headings and subheadings. On this page, write the first paragraph of the paper according to your outline.

_____
_____
_____
_____
_____
_____
_____
_____
_____
_____
_____
_____
_____
_____
_____
_____
_____
_____
_____
_____
_____
_____

Table IC.   Editing Exercise: Word Use

The words or phrases in Column 1 represent common problems in biomedical writing.
In Column 2, write a better expression of the thought.

Column 1—Problems	Column 2—Preferred Word or Phrase
Errors	
The data shows that	_____
Possible contaminated blood	_____
The patient was transfused	_____
The patient took their medication	_____
There was no pathology in the liver	_____
Wordy expressions	
Basic fundamental essentials	_____
In close proximity to	_____
Encourage the patient to ambulate	_____
The subject was cognizant of the study	_____
The vast majority of	_____
Faulty usage	
Free V.D. information, to get it call . . .	_____
One observation mitigated against the diagnosis	_____
Research in presently in progress	_____
The blood pressure gradient between systolic and diastolic	_____
Hopefully, a new treatment will be developed	_____

Table ID.   Editing Exercise: Sentence Structure

Instructions: What is wrong with the sentences in the two paragraphs below? Rewrite
both paragraphs in the space provided.

All the years of training during medical school and the family practice residency and,
indeed, the very concept of family practice as a specialty are focused on a single
moment—the encounter between a patient and the family physician—which
constitutes the wedding of family medicine principles and practice, the rendering of
care by a single family physician to the patient in the context of family.

Table ID *(continued)*

Usually the setting is the physician's office. The scene opens with a telephone call. This is followed by the patient's visit to the office. A dialogue occurs. One human touches another. Accord is reached. Plans are made. This is a drama that has been acted out thousands of times. It has been recorded in scores of civilizations. The ritual of the patient-physician encounter has been with us since before the time of Hippocrates.

Table IE.   Editing Exercise: Revision

Instructions: Revise the following sentence, correcting all errors and making the prose as clear as possible.

This observer believes that, the most common criticism made presently by older practioners are that young graduates have been taught a great deal of information about the mechanism of disease but little relative to the practice of medicine—or to put it in a more blunt fashion, they are too "scientific" and not know how to take appropriate care of patients'.

Hint: The sentence above[a] contains:
   A. Five examples of wordiness
   B. Three examples of word misuse
   C. Two punctuation errors
   D. One misspelling

Location of Errors:

This observer believes that (wordiness), (inappropriate punctuation) the most common criticism made presently (misuse) by older practioners (misspelling) are (misuse) that young graduates have been taught a great deal of information (wordiness) about the mechanisms of disease but little relative to (wordiness) the practice of medicine—or, to put it in a more blunt fashion (wordiness), they are too "scientific" and not (misuse) know how to take appropriate (wordiness) care of patients' (inappropriate possessive).

Original Version:

The most common criticism made at present by older practitioners is that young graduates have been taught a great deal about the mechanism of disease but little about the practice of medicine—or, to put it more bluntly, they are too "scientific" and do not know how to take care of patients.

[a]Adapted (with apologies) from: Peabody F. W. The care of the patient. *JAMA* Vol. 88, pp. 877–882, 1927.

Appendix II

Table IIA. Model Research Protocol[a]

Title Page
    A. Title of study
    B. Principle investigator
    C. Co-investigators
    D. Department chairman
    E. Date submitted
  I. Summary of Proposed Project
    A. Statement of the problem
       1. Purpose of the study
       2. Hypothesis
       3. Questions to be answered
    B. Background
       1. Previous studies/review of the literature
       2. Current status of research
       3. Preliminary work by investigators
    C. Rationale for proposed approach
    D. Significance of study
       1. Importance to medical science
       2. Benefit to patient, if any
    E. Method
       1. Study subjects
          a. Sample size
          b. Eligibility criteria
          c. Classes of subjects excluded
       2. Study design
          a. Procedures

        b. Reporting
        c. Controls
     3. Safeguards
        a. Protection against risk to patients
        b. Protection of confidentiality
        c. Ethical considerations
     4. Data analysis
        a. Data processing
        b. Tests of statistical significance
  F. Project period
     1. Beginning date
     2. Completion date
II. Research Potential
  A. Facilities available
     1. Space: office, clinical, laboratory, or other
     2. Equipment
     3. Supplies
  B. Support from additional sources
     1. In hand
        a. Department funds
        b. Grant, including grant number
        c. Other
     2. Pending—other applications submitted and amounts
     3. Proposed—applications planned to outside agencies
III. Budget   Cost
  A. Equipment (list expensive items by company and catalog
     number) .... $_____
  B. Supplies (list major categories only) .... _____
  C. Services (word processing, computer, other) .... _____
  D. Other expenses .... _____
                                                 Total.... $_____
IV. References
 V. Appendix
  A. Informed Consent Form, which often includes:
     1. Patient record number
     2. Study record number
     3. Nature and purpose of study
     4. Benefit or lack of benefit to subject, if appropriate
     5. Possible untoward effects
     6. Patient's right to refuse to participate
     7. Statement that participation (or refusal to participate) will have no influence on health care now or in the future
     8. Statement that study and informed consent have been explained, with opportunity to ask questions
     9. Signature of subject (or parent/guardian if under 18); date
     10. Signature of investigator who explained study and witnessed signature; date
  B. Report Form(s) or Questionnaire(s)
  C. Other pertinent data, if appropriate
     1. Curriculum vitae of investigator(s)
     2. Correspondence
     3. Reports of prior/pilot studies

---

[a]Adapted from Taylor, R.B. A practical guide to research planning. *Fam. Med.* Vol. 12(6), pp. 25–26, 1980.

Table IIB.   Model Permission Request

Date: _____

Dear Sir:

In the forthcoming book tentatively titled _____
to be published by _____, I would like to
reprint the following material which originally appeared in:

Author(s) _____

Book/Journal/Article Title _____

_____

Specific Material _____

_____

I request your permission to reprint the material specified, with nonexclusive
world rights in the English language, in the forthcoming book and in all future
editions and revisions. Your agreement may be indicated by signing and returning
this letter. We agree that full credit will be given to the author and publisher.

If you do not control these rights in their entirety, please let me know with whom I
should communicate. If permission of the author is also required, please provide
me with an address.

Consideration of this request at your earliest convenience will be much appreciated.

Sincerely,

Please return to: _____

_____

_____

_____

We grant the permission requested on the terms stated in this letter.

by _____

Date: _____

Appendix III

Proofreader's marks are used by authors, editors, and compositors to indicate needed changes in galley and page proofs. Some marks are more or less self-explanatory, such as the symbols to "close up entirely" or to "transpose." Most proofreader marks, however, are a "learned language" and the medical author must keep in mind, for instance, that:

a diagonal line through a capital letter means to print lower case, not to omit the letter;

underlined words set in roman type will be changed to italics; and

"stet" means to leave everything as it was originally printed.

Note that there should always be two marks: one in the text and another in the margin.

If the author is in doubt as to which proofreader mark is appropriate, a clearly written note will always suffice.

Most standard proofreader's marks are listed on pages 214–5.

PROOFREADER'S MARKS

Marginal sign	Mark in text	Meaning	Corrected text
ɣ	Proofreadings	Delete, take out letter or word	Proofreading
e	Legibiljity is	Delete and close up	Legibility is
first	the requirement	Insert marginal addition	the first requirement
‿	of a proof reader's marks.	Close up entirely	of a proofreader's marks.
‿	Symbols should be	Less space	Symbols should be
#	injline with	Add space	in line with
eq.#	the text to which	Space evenly	the text to which
¶	they refer. Place	New paragraph	they refer.
no ¶	marks carefully. Paragraphs may be	No new paragraph	Place marks carefully. Paragraphs may be
□	□ indented one em	Indent one em	indented one em
□□	□□ two ems or (rarely)	Indent two ems	two ems or (rarely)
□□□	□□□ three ems. Head-	Indent three ems	three ems
⌈	⌈ings are flush left	Move to the left	Headings are flush left
⌉	or flush right ▭	Move to the right	or flush right
⌉⌈	⌉ or centered ⌈	Center	or centered
⊔	Mar^ginal marks	Lower to proper position	Marginal marks
⊓	are sep^arated	Raise to proper position	are separated
X	by vertical	Replace defective letter	by vertical
9	lines. The first correction	Invert this letter	lines. The first correction
w.f.	in a line of type	Wrong font; change to proper face	in a line of type
tr.	is beside noted the	Transpose	is noted beside the
?	nearest bend of the line.	Is this correct?	nearest end of the line
Sp.	and the (2nd) next.	Spell out	and the second, next.
	(in this way) both margins	Transfer to position shown by arrow.	both margins are used in
	are used		this way
b.f.	English Finish	Change to boldface type	**English Finish**
b.f. ital.	English Finish	Change to boldface italics	***English Finish***
rom.	*galley* proof	Set in roman type	galley proof
ital.	is laid paper	Set in italics	is *laid* paper

PROOFREADER'S MARKS (continued)

Marginal sign	Mark in text	Meaning	Corrected text
u.c.	Book of type	Set in upper case, or capital	Book of Type
Caps.	Book Papers	Set in large capitals	**BOOK PAPERS**
s.c.	BOOK PAPERS	Change to small capitals	BOOK PAPERS
c.s.c.	Book Papers	Initial large capitals; other letters, small capitals	BOOK PAPERS
l.c.	the first Type	Change to lower case or small letter	the first type
×	baseball player	Broken type	baseball player
Stet	to the editors	Retain crossed out word	to the editors
	Water, HO	Insert inferior figure	Water, H_2O
	$X^2 \div Y^2 = Z$	Insert superior figure	$X^2 \div Y^2 = Z^2$
$\equiv$	printed	Straighten line	printed
‖	The paper	Align type	The paper
	The ink		The ink
	The type		The type
ld.	prepare copy and submit it	Insert lead between lines	prepare copy and submit it
hr.#	PAPER	Hair space between letters	P A P E R
⊙	to the printer	Insert period	to the printer.
⋀	the proof but	Insert comma	the proof, but
; or ;/	excellent it is	Insert semicolon	excellent; it is
: or ⊙	to the following	Insert colon	to the following:
⌄	authors notes	Insert apostrophe	author's notes
⌄/⌄	called caps	Insert quotation marks	called "caps"
-/or =	halftone	Insert hyphen	half-tone
—	Robert Henderson	Insert em dash	—Robert Henderson
–	1939 1940	Insert en dash	1939–1940
?	"Where" she asked.	Insert question mark	"Where?" she asked.
!	"Stop" he cried.	Insert exclamation mark	"Stop!" he cried.
(/)	author see page 2	Insert parentheses	author (see page 2)
[/]	To be continued	Insert brackets	[To be continued]

Appendix IV

Uniform Requirements for Manuscripts Submitted to Biomedical Journals

INTERNATIONAL COMMITTEE OF MEDICAL JOURNAL EDITORS*

In January 1978, a group of editors from some major biomedical journals published in English met in Vancouver, British Columbia, and decided on uniform technical requirements for manuscripts to be submitted to their journals. These requirements, including formats for bibliographic references, were published in three of the journals early in 1979. The Vancouver group evolved into the International Committee of Medical Journal Editors. At the October 1981 meeting of the Committee the requirements were revised slightly and are presented as the main part of this document.

---

*Ole Harlem (*Norwegian Medical Journal*), Edward J. Huth (*Annals of Internal Medicine*), Stephen P. Lock (*British Medical Journal*), Ian Munro (*The Lancet*), Arnold Relman (*The New England Journal of Medicine*), Povl Riis (*Danish Medical Bulletin*), Richard Robinson (*New Zealand Medical Journal*), Andrew Sherrington (*Canadian Medical Association Journal*), M. Therese Southgate (*Journal of the American Medical Association*), Ilka Vartiovaara (*Finnish Medical Journal*).

Over 150 journals have now agreed to receive manuscripts prepared in accordance with these requirements. It is important to emphasize what these requirements imply and what they do not.

First, if authors prepare their manuscripts in the style specified in these requirements, editors will not return manuscripts for changes in details of style. Even so, manuscripts may be altered by journals to conform with details of their own publication styles.

Second, the requirements are instructions to authors on how to prepare manuscripts, not to editors on publication style.

Thirdly, authors sending manuscripts to a participating journal should not try to prepare them in accordance with the individual publication style of that journal but should follow the "Uniform Requirements for Manuscripts Submitted to Biomedical Journals."

Nevertheless authors *must also* follow the instructions to authors in the journal as to what topics are suitable for that journal and the types of papers that may be submitted (for example, original articles, reviews, case reports). In addition, the journal's instructions are likely to contain other requirements unique to that journal, such as number of copies of manuscripts, acceptable languages, length of articles, and approved abbreviations besides those listed in this document.

The cooperating journals are expected to state in their instructions to authors that their requirements are in accordance with "Uniform Requirements for Manuscripts Submitted to Biomedical Journals."

This document will be revised at intervals. Inquiries and comments from Central and North America about these requirements should be sent to Edward J. Huth, M.D., *Annals of Internal Medicine*, 4200 Pine Street, Philadelphia, PA 19104, USA; those from other regions should be sent to Stephen P. Lock, F.R.C.P., *British Medical Journal*, British Medical Association, Tavistock Square, London WC1H 9JR, United Kingdom.

Summary of Requirements

Type the manuscript double spaced, including title page, abstract, text, acknowledgments, references, tables, and legends.

Source: Annals of Internal Medicine. 1982;96 (Part 1):766–771. Reprinted with permission.

Each manuscript component should begin on a new page, in the following sequence.

Title page

Abstract and key words

Text

Acknowledgments

References

Tables: each table, complete with title and footnotes, on a separate page

Legends for illustrations

Illustrations must be good-quality, unmounted glossy prints usually 127 by 173 mm (5 by 7 in.) but no larger than 203 by 254 mm (8 × 10 in.).

Submit the required number of copies of manuscript and figures (*see* journal's instructions) in a heavy-paper envelope. The submitted manuscript should be accompanied by a covering letter, as described under "Submission of Manuscripts," and permissions to reproduce previously published materials or to use illustrations that may identify human subjects.

Follow the journal's instructions for transfer of copyright. Authors should keep copies of everything submitted.

Prior and Duplicate Publication

Most journals do not wish to consider for publication a paper on work that already has been reported in a published paper, or is described in a paper submitted or accepted for publication elsewhere. This policy does not usually preclude consideration of a manuscript that has been rejected by another journal or of a complete report that follows publication of a preliminary report, usually in the form of an abstract. When submitting a manuscript, an author should always make a full statement to the editor about all submissions and prior reports that might be regarded as prior or duplicate publication of the same or very similar work. Copies of such material should be included with the submitted manuscript to help the editor decide how to deal with the matter.

Preparation of Manuscript

Type the manuscript on white bond paper, 216 × 279 mm (8½ × 11 in.) or ISO A4 (212 × 297 mm), with margins of at least 25 mm (1 in.) Type only on one side of the paper. Use double spacing throughout, including title page, abstract, text, acknowledgments, references, tables, and legends for illustrations. Begin each of the following sections on separate pages: title page, abstract and key words, text, acknowledgments, references, individual tables, and legends. Number pages consecutively, beginning with the title page. Type the page number in the upper right-hand corner of each page.

Title Page

The title page should carry (1) the title of the article, which should be concise but informative; (2) a short running head or footline of no more than 40 characters (count letters and spaces) placed at the foot of the title page and identified; (3) first name, middle initial, and last name of each author, with highest academic degree(s); (4) name of department(s) and institution(s) to which the work should be attributed; (5) disclaimers, if any; (6) name and address of author responsible for correspondence about the manuscript; (7) name and address of author to whom requests for reprints should be addressed, or statement that reprints will not be available from the author; (8) the source(s) of support in the form of grants, equipment, drugs , or all of these.

Abstract and Key Words

The second page should carry an abstract of no more than 150 words. The abstract should state the purposes of the study or investigation, basic procedures (study subjects or experimental animals; observational and analytic methods), main findings (give specific data and their statistical significance, if possible), and the principal conclusions. Emphasize new and important aspects of the study or observations. Use only approved abbreviations (*see* Commonly Used Approved Abbreviations, elsewhere in this document).

Below the abstract, provide, and identify as such, 3 to 10 key words or short phrases that will assist indexers in cross-indexing your article and that may be published with the abstract. Use terms from the Medical Subject Headings list from *Index Medicus* when possible.

Text

The text of observational and experimental articles is usually—but not necessarily—divided into sections with the headings Introduction, Methods, Results, and Discussion. Long articles may need subheadings within some sections to clarify their content, especially the Results and Discussion sections. Other types of articles such as case reports, reviews, and editorials are likely to need other formats, and authors should consult individual journals for further guidance.

Introduction. Clearly state the purpose of the article. Summarize the rationale for the study or observation. Give only strictly pertinent references, and do not review the subject extensively.

Methods. Describe your selection of the observational or experimental subjects (patients or experimental animals, including controls) clearly. Identify the methods, apparatus (manufacturer's name and address in parentheses), and procedures in sufficient detail to allow other workers to reproduce the results. Give references to established methods, including statistical methods; provide references and brief descriptions for methods that have been published but are not well known; describe new or substantially modified methods, give reasons for using them, and evaluate their limitations.

When reporting experiments on human subjects, indicate whether the procedures followed were in accordance with the ethical standards of the committee on human experimentation of the institution in which the experiments were done or in accordance with the Helsinki Declaration of 1975. When reporting experiments on animals, indicate whether the institution's or the National Research Council's guide for the care and use of laboratory animals was followed. Identify precisely all drugs and chemicals used, including generic name(s), dosage(s), and route(s) of administration. Do not use patients' names, initials, or hospital numbers.

Include numbers of observations and the statistical significance of the findings when appropriate. Detailed statistical analyses, mathematical derivations, and the like may sometimes be suitably presented in the form of one or more appendixes.

Results. Present your results in logical sequence in the text, tables, and illustrations. Do not repeat in the text all the data in the tables, illustrations, or both; emphasize or summarize only important observations.

Discussion. Emphasize the new and important aspects of the study and conclusions that follow from them. Do not repeat in detail data given in the Results section. Include in the Discussion the implications of the findings and their limitations and relate the observations to other relevant studies. Link the conclusions with the goals of the study but avoid unqualified statements and conclusions not completely supported by your data. Avoid claiming priority and alluding to work that has not been completed. State new hypotheses when warranted, but clearly label them as such. Recommendations, when appropriate, may be included.

Acknowledgments

Acknowledge only persons who have made substantive contributions to the study. Authors are responsible for obtaining written permission from persons acknowledged by name because readers may infer their endorsement of the data and conclusions.

References

Number references consecutively in the order in which they are first mentioned in the text. Identify references in text, tables, and legends by arabic numerals (in parentheses). References cited *only* in tables or in legends to figures should be numbered in accordance with a sequence established by the first identification in the text of the particular table or illustration.

Use the style of the examples below, which are based on the formats used by the U.S. National Library of Medicine in *Index Medicus.*

The titles of journals should be abbreviated according to the style used in *Index Medicus*. A list of abbreviated names of frequently cited journals is given near the end of this document; for others, consult "List of the Journals Indexed," printed annually in the January issue of *Index Medicus.*

Try to avoid using abstracts as references; "unpublished observations" and "personal communications" may not be used as references, although references to written, not verbal, communications may be inserted (in parentheses) in the text. Include among the references manuscripts accepted but not yet published; designate the journal followed by "in press" (in parentheses). Information from manuscripts submitted but not yet accepted should be cited in the text as "unpublished observations" (in parentheses).

The references must be verified by the author(s) against the original documents.

Examples of correct forms of references are given below.

Journals

(1) Standard Journal Article (List all authors when six or less; when seven or more, list only first three and add et al.)
   You CH, Lee KY, Chey RY, Menguy R. Electrogastrographic study of patients with unexplained nausea, bloating and vomiting. Gastroenterology 1980;79:311–4.

(2) Corporate Author
   The Royal Marsden Hospital Bone-Marrow Transplantation Team. Failure of syngeneic bone marrow graft without preconditioning in post-hepatitis marrow aplasia. Lancet 1977;2:242–4.

(3) No Author Given
   Anonymous. Coffee drinking and cancer of the pancreas [Editorial]. Br Med J 1981;283:628.

(4) Journal Supplement
   Mastri AR. Neuropathy of diabetic neurogenic bladder. Ann Intern Med 1980;92(2 Pt 2):316–8.

   Frumin AM, Nussbaum J, Esposito M. Functional asplenia: demonstration of splenic activity by bone marrow scan [Abstract]. Blood 1979;54(suppl 1):26a.

(5) Journal Paginated by Issue
   Seaman WB. The case of the pancreatic pseudocyst. Hosp Pract 1981;16(Sep):24–5.

Books and Other Monographs

(6) Personal Author(s)
     Eisen HN. Immunology: an introduction to molecular and cellular principles of the immune response. 5th ed. New York: Harper and Row, 1974:406.

(7) Editor, Compiler, Chairman as Author
     Dausset J, Colombani J, eds. Histocompatibility testing 1972. Copenhagen: Munksgaard, 1973:12–8.

(8) Chapter in a Book
     Weinstein L, Swartz MN. Pathogenic properties of invading microorganisms. In: Sodeman WA Jr, Sodeman WA, eds. Pathologic physiology: mechanisms of disease. Philadelphia: WB Saunders, 1974:457–72.

(9) Published Proceedings Paper
     DuPont B. Bone marrow transplantation in severe combined immunodeficiency with an unrelated MLC compatible donor. In: White HJ, Smith R, eds. Proceedings of the third annual meeting of the International Society for Experimental Hematology. Houston: International Society for Experimental Hematology, 1974:44–6.

(10) Monograph in a Series
     Hunninghake GW, Gadek JE, Szapiel SV, et al. The human alveolar macrophage. In: Harris CC, ed. Cultured human cells and tissues in biomedical research. New York: Academic Press, 1980:54–6. (Stoner GD, ed. Methods and perspectives in cell biology; vol 1).

(11) Agency Publication
     Ranofsky AL. Surgical operations in short-stay hospitals: United States—1975. Hyattsville, Maryland: National Center for Health Statistics, 1978; DHEW publication no. (PHS) 78-1785. (Vital and health statistics; series 13; no 34).

(12) Dissertation or Thesis
     Cairns RB. Infrared spectroscopic studies of solid oxygen [Dissertation]. Berkeley, California: University of California, 1965. 156 p.

Other Articles

(13) Newspaper Article
     Shaffer RA. Advances in chemistry are starting to unlock mysteries of the brain: discoveries could help cure alcoholism and insomnia, explain mental illness. How the messengers work. Wall Street Journal 1977 Aug 12:1(col 1), 10(col 1).

(14) Magazine Article
     Roueché B. Annals of medicine: the Santa Claus culture. The New Yorker 1971 Sep 4:66–81.

Tables

Type each table on a separate sheet; remember to double space. Do not submit tables as photographs. Number tables consecutively and supply a brief title for each. Give each column a short or abbreviated heading. Place explanatory matter in footnotes, not in the heading. Explain in footnotes all nonstandard abbreviations that are used in each table. For footnotes, use the following symbols, in this sequence: *, †, ‡, §, ||, ¶, **, † †....

Identify statistical measures of variations such as standard deviation and standard error of the mean.

Do not use internal horizontal and vertical rules.

Cite each table in the text in consecutive order.

If you use data from another published or unpublished source, obtain permission and acknowledge fully.

The use of too many tables in relation to the length of the text may produce difficulties in the layout of pages. Examine issues of the journal to which you plan to submit your manuscript to estimate how many tables can be used per 1000 words of text.

The editor, on accepting a manuscript, may recommend that additional tables containing important backup data too extensive to publish be deposited with the National Auxiliary Publications Service or made available by the author(s). In that event, an appropriate statement will be added to the text. Submit such tables for consideration with the manuscript.

Illustrations

Submit the required number of complete sets of figures. Figures should be professionally drawn and photographed; freehand or typewritten lettering is unacceptable. Instead of *original* drawings, roentgenograms, and other material, send sharp, glossy black-and-white photographic prints, usually 127 × 173 mm (5 × 7 in.) but no larger than 203 × 254 mm (8 × 10 in.). Letters, numbers, and symbols should be clear and even throughout, and of sufficient size that when reduced for publication each item will still be legible. Titles and detailed explanations belong in the legends for illustrations, not on the illustrations themselves.

Each figure should have a label pasted on its back indicating the number of the figure, the names of the authors, and the top of the figure. Do not write on the back of the figures, mount them on cardboard, or scratch or mar them using paper clips. Do not bend figures.

Photomicrographs must have internal scale markers. Symbols, arrows, or letters used in the photomicrographs should contrast with the background.

If photographs of persons are used, either the subjects must not be identifiable or their pictures must be accompanied by written permission to use the photograph.

Cite each figure in the text in consecutive order. If a figure has been published, acknowledge the original source and submit written permission from the copyright holder to reproduce the material. Permission is required, *regardless of authorship or publisher*, except for documents in the public domain.

For illustrations in color, supply color negatives or positive transparencies and, when necessary, accompanying drawings marked to indicate the region to be reproduced; in addition, send two positive color prints to assist editors in making recommendations. Some journals publish illustrations in color only if the author pays for the extra cost.

Legends for Illustrations

Type legends for illustrations double spaced, starting on a separate page, with arabic numerals corresponding to the illustrations. When symbols, arrows, numbers, or letters are used to identify parts of the illustrations, identify and explain each one clearly in the legend. Explain internal scale and identify method of staining in photomicrographs.

Units of Measurement

Measurements of length, height, weight, and volume should be reported in metric units (meter, kilogram, liter) or their decimal multiples.

Temperatures should be given in degrees Celsius. Blood pressures should be given in millimetres of mercury. Other measurements should be reported in the units in which they were made.

In most countries the International System of Units (SI) is standard or is becoming so. Journals may use these units or convert them to other units according to their editorial policies. Editors may request that alternative units (SI or non-SI units) be added by the author before publication of the paper.

Abbreviations and Symbols

Use only standard abbreviations (*see* below for lists of commonly used abbreviations). Consult the following sources for additional abbreviations: (1) CBE Style Manual Committee. Council of Biology Editors style manual: a guide for authors, editors, and publishers in the biological sciences. 4th ed. Arlington, Virginia: Council of Biology Editors, 1978; and (2) O'Connor M, Woodford FP. Writing scientific papers in English: an ELSE-Ciba Foundation guide for authors. Amsterdam: Elsevier-Excerpta Medica, 1975. Avoid abbreviations in the title. The full term for which an abbreviation stands should precede its first use in the text unless it is a standard unit of measurement.

Submission of Manuscripts

Mail the required number of manuscript copies in a heavy-paper envelope, enclosing the manuscript copies and figures in cardboard, if necessary, to prevent bending of photographs during mail handling. Place photographs and transparencies in a separate heavy-paper envelope.

Manuscripts should be accompanied by a covering letter from the author who will be responsible for correspondence regarding the manuscript. The covering letter should contain a statement that the manuscript has been seen and approved by all authors. The letter should give any additional information that may be helpful to the editor, such as the type of article the manuscript represents in the particular journal, information on prior or duplicate publication or submission of any part of the work, and whether the author(s) will be willing to meet the cost of reproducing color illustrations. Include copies of any permissions needed to reproduce published material or to use illustrations of identifiable subjects.

ABBREVIATIONS OF NAMES OF FREQUENTLY CITED JOURNALS; PARTICIPATING JOURNALS

The journals listed below by abbreviated title are those covered by *Abridged Index Medicus* and additional journals participating in the Uniform Requirements agreement. Participating journals are marked by an asterisk.

Acta Paediatr Scand*
Activox*
AJR*
Am Fam Physician*
Am Heart J
Am J Cardiol*
Am J Clin Nutr*
Am J Clin Pathol
Am J Dis Child*
Am J Epidemiol*
Am J Hosp Pharm*
Am J Hum Genet*
Am J Med*
Am J Med Sci
Am J Nurs
Am J Obstet Gynecol
Am J Ophthalmol
Am J Pathol*
Am J Phys Med
Am J Psychiatry*
Am J Public Health*
Am J Surg*

Am J Trop Med Hyg
Am Rev Respir Dis*
Am Surg*
Anaesthesia*
Anaesth Intensive Care*
Anesth Analg (Cleve)*
Anesthesiology
Ann Clin Biochem*
Ann Clin Lab Sci*
Ann Intern Med*
Ann Otol Rhinol Laryngol*
Ann R Coll Phys Surg Can*
Ann R Col Surg Engl*
Ann Rheum Dis*
Ann Surg*
Ann Thorac Surg*
Ann Trop Paediatr*
Arch Dermatol*
Arch Dis Child*
Arch Environ Health
Arch Gen Psychiatry*
Arch Intern Med*

Arch Invest Med (Mex)*
Arch Neurol*
Arch Ophthalmol*
Arch Otolaryngol*
Arch Pathol Lab Med*
Arch Phys Med Rehabil
Arch Surg*
Ariz Med*
Arteriosclerosis*
Arthritis Rheum
Aust Fam Physician*
Aust J Derm*
Aust J Hosp Pham*
Aust J Ophthalmol*
Aust NZ J Med*
Aust NZ J Surg*
Aust Paediatr J*
Bibl Laeger*
Blood
Bol Med Hosp Infant Mex*
Bordeaux Med*
Brain
Brain Develop*
Br Heart J*
Br Homeopath J*
Br J Ind Med*
Br J Obstet Gynaecol
Br J Ophthalmol*
Br J Pain*
Br J Radiol
Br J Surg*
Br J Vener Dis*
Br Med J*
Bull Med Libr Assoc*
Bull WHO*
CA
Cancer
Can J Public Health*
Can J Surg*
Can Med Assoc J*
Cardiovasc Res*
Cephalalgia*
Chest*
Chron Dis Can*
Circulation*
Clin Chem Acta*
Clin Invest Med*
Clin Orthop
Clin Pediatr (Phila)*
Clin Pharmacol Ther
Clin Prevent Dent*
Clin Toxicol
Community Med*
Crit Care Med
Cuad Hosp Clin*

Curr Concepts Hyperten Cardiovasc Dis*
Curr Probl Surg
Dan Med Bull*
Diabetes
Dig Dis Sci
DM
Drug Intell Clin Pharm*
Endocrinology
Eur Heart J*
Eur J Cancer*
Eur J Clin Invest*
Eur J Resp Dis*
Eur J Rheum Inflam*
Fam Med Teacher*
Fin Med J*
Gastroenterology*
Gastrointest Endosc*
Geriatrics*
Gut*
Hawaii Med J*
Heart Lung
Hospitals
Hosp Pharm*
Hosp Pract
Iatriki*
Indian J Dermatol Venereol Leprol*
Int J Epidemiol*
Int J Pediatr Nephrol*
Int Rehab Med*
J Allergy Clin Immunol*
JAMA*
J Am Diet Assoc
J Bone Joint Surg (Am)
J Bone Joint Surg (Br)
J Cardiovasc Surg*
J Chronic Dis*
J Clin Endocrinol Metab
J Clin Gastroenterol*
J Clin Invest
J Clin Pathol*
J Epidemiol Community Health*
J Fac Med (Baghdad)*
J Fam Pract
J Gerontol
J Hong Kong Med Technol Assoc*
J Immunol
J Irish Coll Physicians Surg*
J Infect Dis
J Lab Clin Med*
J Laryngol Otol
J Manipul Physiol Therap*
J Matern Child Health*
J Med Ethics*
J Med Educ
J Med Genet*

J Natl Cancer Inst*
J Nephrol*
J Nerv Ment Dis
J Neurol Neurosurg Psychiatry*
J Neurosurg
J Nucl Med Technol*
J Nurs Adm
J Oral Surg
J Pediatr
J Psychosom Res*
J R Army Med Corps*
J R Coll Physicians Lond*
J R Coll Surg Edinb*
J R Nav Med Ser*
J thorac Cardiovasc Surg
J Trauma
J Urol
J Vivekananda Inst Med Sci*
Lakartidningen*
Lancet*
Lepr Rev*
Malay J Pathol*
Matern Child Health*
Mayo Clin Proc
Med Care*
Med Clin (Barc)*
Med Clin North Am
Medicine (Baltimore)
Medicine (Oxford)*
Med J Aust*
Med Lab Sci*
Med Lett Drugs Ther
Med Pediatr Oncol*
Mt Sinai J Med*
N Carolina Med J*
N Doct*
Ned Tijdschr Geneeskd*
N Engl J Med*
Neurology (NY)*
Newfoundland Med Assoc J*
Niger Med J*
Nord Med*
No To Hattatsu*
Nurs Clin North Am
Nursing*
Nurs Outlook
Nurs Res
NZ Fam Physician*
NZ Med J*
NZ J Med Lab Technol*
Obstet Gynecol
Ophthalmology*
Orthop Clin North Am

Orthopt J Aust*
Otolaryngol Head Neck Surg*
Papua New Guinea Med J*
Pathology*
Pediatr Clin North Am
Pediatrics
Periton Dialys Bull*
Pharmacotherapy*
Physician Sports Med*
Phys Ther
Plast Reconstr Surg
PM*
Postgrad Doct-Africa*
Postgrad Doct-Asia*
Postgrad Doct-Middle East*
Postgrad Med*
Postgrad Med J*
Prog Cardiovasc Dis
Public Health*
Public Health Pap*
Public Health Rep
Quart J Med*
Radiol Clin North Am
Radiology*
Rev Esp Rheumatol*
Rev Med Chil*
Rev Med IMSS*
Rheumatol Rehabil
S Afr Med J*
Scand J Respir Dis*
Sex Transm Dis*
South Med J*
Sri Lankan Farm Physician*
Surg Clin North Am
Surgery
Surg Gynecol Obstet
Swed Med J*
Thorax*
Thromb Haemost*
Tidsskr Nor Laegeforen*
Transfusion*
Trop Gastroenterol*
Ugeskr Laeger*
Ulster Med J*
Undersea Biomed Res*
Urol Clin North Am
Vet Radiol*
WHO Chron*
WHO Monogr Ser*
WHO Tech Rep Ser*
World Health Stat Q*
World Med J*
Yale J Biol Med*

Commonly Used Approved Abbreviations

Standard Units of Measurement

ampere	A	centi- (10^{-2})	c
ångström	Å	milli- (10^{-3})	m
barn	b	micro- (10^{-6})	μ
candela	cd	nano- (10^{-9})	n
coulomb	C	pico- (10^{-12})	p
counts per minute	cpm	femto- (10^{-15})	f
counts per second	cps	atto- (10^{-18})	a
curie	Ci		
degree Celsius	°C	*Stastical Terms*	
disintegration per minute	dpm	correlation coefficient	r
disintegration per second	dps	degrees of freedom	df
electron volt	eV	mean	x̄
equivalent	Eq	not significant	NS
farad	F	number of observations	n
gauss	G	probability	p
gram	g	standard deviation	SD
henry	H	standard error of the mean	SEM
hertz	Hz	"Student's" t test	t test
hour	h	variance ratio	F
international unit	IU		
joule	J		
kelvin	K	*Others*	
kilogram	kg	adenosinediphosphatase	ADPase
liter, litre	l or L	adenosine 5'-diphosphate	
meter, metre	m	(adenosine diphosphate)	ADP
minute	min	adenosine 5'-monophosphate	
molar	M	(adenosine monophosphate,	
mole	mol	adenylic acid)	AMP
newton	N	adenosine triphosphatase	ATPase
normal (concentration)	N	adenosine 5'-triphosphate	
ohm	Ω	(adenosine triphosphate)	ATP
osmole	osmol	adrenocorticotropic hormone	
pascal	Pa	(adrenocorticotropin)	ACTH
revolutions per minute	rpm	bacille Calmette-Guérin	BCG
second	s	basal metabolic rate	BMR
square centimetre	cm^2	body temperature, pressure,	
volt	V	and saturated	BTPS
watt	W	central nervous system	CNS
week	wk	coenzyme A	coA
year	yr	deoxyribonucleic acid	
		(deoxyribonucleate)	DNA
Combining Prefixes		dihydroxyphenethylamine	dopamine
tera- (10^{12})	T	electrocardiogram	ECG
giga- (10^{9})	G	electroencephalogram	EEG
mega- (10^{6})	M	enteric cytopathogenic human	
kilo- (10^{3})	k	orphan (virus)	ECHO
hecto- (10^{2})	h	ethyl	Et
deca- (10^{1})	da	ethylenediaminetetraacetate	EDTA
deci- (10^{-1})	d	gas-liquid chromatography	GLC

guanosine 5′-monophosphate (guanosine monophosphate, guanylic acid)	GMP	radiation (ionizing, absorbed dose)	rad
hemoglobin	Hb	respiratory quotient	RQ
logarithm (to base 10; common logarithm)	log	specific gravity	sp gr
		standard atmosphere	atm
logarithm, natural	ln	standard temperature and pressure	STP
methyl	Me	ultraviolet	uv
Michaelis constant	K_m	volume	vol
negative logarithm of hydrogen ion activity	pH	volume ratio (volume per volume)	vol/vol
partial pressure of CO_2	P_{CO_2}	weight	wt
partial pressure of O_2	P_{O_2}	weight per volume	wt/vol
per	/	weight ratio (weight per weight)	wt/wt
percent	%		

Appendix V

Copyright Basics[a]

On January 1, 1978,the Copyright Act of 1976 (title 17 of the United States Code) came into effect. This general revision of the copyright law of the United States, the first such revision since 1909, makes important changes in our copyright system and generally, but not entirely, supersedes the previous Federal copyright statute. For highlights of the overall changes in the copyright law, request Circular R99 from the Copyright Office.

What Copyright Is

Copyright is a form of protection provided by the laws of the United States (title 17, U.S. Code) to the authors of "original works of authorship" including literary, dramatic, musical, artistic, and certain other intellectual works. This protection is available to both published and unpublished works. Section 106 of the Copyright Act generally gives the owner of copyright the exclusive right to do and to authorize others to do the following:

to reproduce the copyrighted work in copies or phonorecords;

to prepare derivative works based upon the copyrighted work;

[a]Source Circular R1, U.S. Government Printing Office: 1980-311-426/5

to distribute copies or phonorecords of the copyrighted work to the public by sale or other transfer of ownership, or by rental, lease, or lending;

to perform the copyrighted work publicly, in the case of literary, musical, dramatic, and choreographic works, pantomimes, and motion pictures and other audiovisual works, and

to display the copyrighted work publicly in the case of literary, musical, dramatic, and choreographic, or sculptural works, including the individual images of a motion picture or other audiovisual work.

It is illegal for anyone to violate any of the rights provided to the owner of copyright by the Act. These rights, however, are not unlimited in scope. Sections 107 through 118 of the Copyright Act establish limitations on these rights. In some cases, these limitations are specified exemptions from copyright liability. One major limitation is the doctrine of "fair use," which is now given a statutory basis by section 107 of the Act. In other instances, the limitation takes the form of a "compulsory license" under which certain limited uses of copyrighted works are permitted upon payment of specified royalties and compliance with statutory conditions. For further information about the limitations of any of these rights, consult the Copyright Act or write to the Copyright Office.

Who Can Claim Copyright

Copyright protection subsists from the time the work is created in fixed form; that is, it is an incident of the process of authorship. The copyright in the work of authorship **immediately** becomes the property of the author who created it. Only the author or those deriving their rights through the author can rightfully claim copyright.

In the case of works made for hire, the employer and not the employee is presumptively considered the author. Section 101 of the copyright statute defines a "work made for hire" as:

(1) a work prepared by an employee within the scope of his or her employment; or
(2) a work specially ordered or commissioned for use as a contribution to a collective work, as a part of a motion picture or other audiovisual work, as a translation, as a supplementary work, as a compilation, as an instructional text, as a test, as answer material for a test, or as an atlas, if the parties expressly agree in a written instrument signed by them that the work shall be considered a work made for hire. . . .

The authors of a joint work are co-owners of the copyright in the work, unless there is an agreement to the contrary.

Copyright in each separate contribution to a periodical or other collective work is distinct from copyright in the collective work as a whole and vests initially with the author of the contribution.

Two General Principles

Mere ownership of a book, manuscript, painting, or any other copy or phonorecord does not give the possessor the copyright. The law provides that transfer of ownership of any material object that embodies a protected work does not of itself convey any rights in the copyright.

Minors may claim copyright, but state laws may regulate the business dealings involving copyrights owned by minors. For information on relevant state laws, it would be well to consult an attorney.

Copyright and National Origin of the Work

Copyright protection is available for all unpublished works, regardless of the citizenship or domicile of the author.

Published works are eligible for copyright protection in the U.S. if any one of the following conditions is met:

On the date of first publication, one or more of the authors is a national or domiciliary of the United States or of a country that is a party to a copyright treaty to which the U.S. is also a party, or is a stateless person whatever that person may be domiciled; or

The work is first published in the United States or in a foreign nation that, on the date of first publication, is a party to the Universal Copyright Convention.

For a list of countries which maintain copyright relations with the United States, write to the Copyright Office and ask for Circular R38a.

What Works Are Protected

Copyright protection exists for "original works of authorship" when they become fixed in a tangible form of expression. The fixation does not need to be directly perceptible, so long as it may be communicated with the aid of a machine or device. Copyrightable works include the following categories:

(1) literary works;
(2) musical works, including any accompanying words;
(3) dramatic works, including any accompanying music;
(4) pantomimes and choreographic works;

(5) pictorial, graphic, and sculptural works;
(6) motion pictures and other audiovisual works; and
(7) sound recordings.

This list is illustrative and is not meant to exhaust the categories of copyrightable works. These categories should be viewed quite broadly so that, for example, computer programs and most "compilations" are registrable as "literary works"; maps and architectural blueprints are registrable as "pictorial, graphic, and sculptural works."

What Is Not Protected by Copyright

Several categories of material are generally not eligible for statutory copyright protection. These include among others:

Works that have *not* been fixed in a tangible form of expression. For example: choreographic works which have not been notated or recorded, or improvisational speeches or performances that have not been written or recorded.

Titles, names, short phrases, and slogans; familiar symbols or designs; mere variations of typographic ornamentation, lettering, or coloring; mere listings of ingredients or contents.

Ideas, procedures, methods, systems, processes, concepts, principles, discoveries, or devices, as distinguished from a description, explanation, or illustration.

Works consisting *entirely* of information that is common property and containing no original authorship. For example: standard calendars, height and weight charts, tape measures and rules, and lists or tables taken from public documents or other common sources.

How To Secure a Copyright

Copyright Secured Automatically upon Creation

The way in which copyright protection is secured under the new law is frequently misunderstood. No publication or registration or other action in the Copyright Office is required to secure copyright under the new law, unlike the old law, which required either publication with the copyright notice or registration in the Copyright Office (see NOTE below). There are, however, certain definite advantages to registration (later discussed).

Under the new law, copyright is secured *automatically* when the work is created, and a work is "created" when it is fixed in a copy or phonorecord for the first time. In general, "copies" are material objects from which a work can be read or visually perceived either directly or with the aid of a machine or device, such as books, manuscripts, sheet music, film, videotape, or microfilm. "Phonorecords" are material objects embodying fixations of sounds (excluding, by statutory definition, motion picture soundtracks), such as audio tapes and phonograph disks. Thus, for example, a song (the "work") can be fixed in sheet music ("copies") or in phonograph disks ("phonorecords"), or both.

If a work is prepared over a period of time, the part of the work existing in fixed form on a particular date constitutes the created work as of that date.

NOTE: Before 1978, statutory copyright was generally secured by the act of publication with notice of copyright, assuming compliance with all other relevant statutory conditions. Works in the public domain on January 1, 1978 (for example, works published without satisfying all conditions for securing statutory copyright under the Copyright Act of 1909) remain in the public domain under the current Act.

Statutory copyright could also be secured before 1978 by the act of registration in the case of certain unpublished works and works eligible for ad interim copyright. The current Act automatically extends to full term copyright (section 304 sets the term) for all works in which ad interim copyright was subsisting or was capable of being secured on December 31, 1977.

Publication

Publication is no longer the key to obtaining statutory copyright as it was under the Copyright Act of 1909. However, publication remains important to copyright owners.

The Copyright Act defines publication as follows:

> "Publication" is the distribution of copies or phonorecords of a work to the public by sale or other transfer of ownership, or by rental, lease, or lending. The offering to distribute copies or phonorecords to a group of persons for purposes of further distribution, public performance, or public display, constitutes publication. A public performance of display of a work does not of itself constitute publication.

A further discussion of the definition of "publication" can be found in the legislative history of the Act. The legislative reports define "to the public" as distribution to persons under no explicit or implicit restrictions with respect to disclosure of the contents. The reports state that the definition makes it clear that the sale of phonorecords constitutes publication of the underlying work, for example, the musical, dramatic, or literary work embodied in a phonorecord. The reports also state that it is clear that any form or disseemination in which the material object does not change hands, for examle, performances or displays on television, is *not* a publication no matter how many people are exposed to the work. However, when copies or phonorecords are offered for sale or lease to a group of wholesalers, broadcasters, or motion picture theaters, publication does take place if the purpose is further distribution, public performance, or public display.

Publication is an important concept in the copyright law because upon publication, several significant consequences follow. Among these are:

When a work is published, all published copies should bear a notice of copyright. (See discussion below of "notice of copyright.")

Works that are published with notice of copyright in the U.S. are subject to mandatory deposit with the Library of Congress. (See subsequent discussion on "mandatory deposit.")

Publication of a work can affect the limitations on the exclusive rights of the copyright owner that are set forth in sections 107 through 118 of the law.

The year of publication is used in determining the duration of copyright protection for anonymous and pseudonymous works (when the author's identity is not revealed in the records of the Copyright Office) and for works made for hire.

Deposit requirements for registration of published works differ from those for registration of unpublished works.

Notice of Copyright

When a work is published under the authority of the copyright owner, a notice of copyright should be placed on all publicly distributed copies and on all publicly distributed phonorecords of sound recordings. This notice is required even on works published outside of the United States. Failure to comply with the notice requirement can result in the loss of certain additional rights otherwise available to the copyright owner.

The use of the copyright notice is the responsibility of the copyright owner and does not require advance permission from, or registration with, the Copyright Office.

Form of Notice for Visually Perceptible Copies

The notice for visually perceptible copies should contain the following three elements:

The symbol © (the letter C in a circle), or the word "Copyright," or the abbreviation "Copr."; and

The year of first publication of the work. In the case of cornpilations or derivative works incorporating previously published material, the year date of first publication of the compilation or derivative work is sufficient. The year date may be omitted where a pictorial, graphic, or sculptural work, with accompanying textual matter, if any, is reproduced in or on greeting cards, postcards, stationery, jewelry, dolls, toys, or any useful article; and

The name of the owner of copyright in the work, or an abbreviation by which the name can be recognized, or a generally known alternative designation of the owner.

Example: © John Doe 1980

The "C in a circle" notice is required only on "visually perceptible copies." Certain kinds of works, for example, musical, dramatic, and literary works, may be fixed not in "copies" but by means of sound in an audio recording. Since audio recordings such as audio tapes and phonograph disks are "phonorecords" and not "copies," there is no requirement that the phonorecrod bear a "C in a circle" notice to protect the underlying musical, dramatic, or literary work that is recorded.

Form of Notice for Phonorecords of Sound Recordings

The copyright notice for phonorecords of sound recordings* has somewhat different requirements. The notice appearing on phonorecords should contain the following three elements:

The symbol ℗ (the letter P in a circle); and

The year of first publication of the sound recording; and

The name of the owner of copyright in the sound recording, or an abbreviation by which the name can be recognized, or a generally known alternative designation of the owner. If the producer of the sound recording is named on the phonorecord labels or containers, and if no other name appears in conjunction with the notice, the producer's name shall be considered a part of the notice.

---

*Sound recordings are defined as "works that result from the fixation of a series of musical, spoken, or other sounds, but not including the sounds accompanying a motion picture or other audiovisual work, regardless of the nature of the material objects, such as disks, tapes, or other phonorecords, in which they are embodied."

Example: ℗ John Doe 1980

NOTE: Because of problems that might result in some cases from the use of variant forms of the notice, any form of the notice other than these given here should not be used without first seeking legal advice.

Position of Notice

The notice should be affixed to copies or phonorecords of the work in such a manner and location as to "give reasonable notice of the claim of copyright." The notice on phonorecords may appear on the surface of the phonorecord or on the phonorecord label or container, provided the manner of placement and location gives reasonable notice of the claim. The three elements of the notice should ordinarily appear together on the copies or phonorecords. For further information about methods of affixation of the notice, write to the Copyright Office.

Unpublished Works

The copyright notice is not required on unpublished works. To avoid an inadvertent publication without notice, however, it may be advisable for the author or other owner of the copyright to affix notices to any copies or phonorecords which leave his or her control.

Effect of Omission of the Notice or of Error in the Name or Date

Unlike the law in effect before 1978, the new Copyright Act, in sections 405 and 406, provides procedures for correcting errors and omissions of the copyright notice on works published on or after January 1, 1978.

In general, the omission or error does not automatically invalidate the copyright in a work if registration for the work has been made before or is made within 5 years after the publication without notice, and a reasonable effort is made to add the notice to all copies or phonorecords that are distributed to the public in the United States after the omission has been discovered.

NOTE: Before 1978, the copyright law required, as a condition for copyright protection, that all copies published with the authorization of the copyright owner bear a proper notice. If a work was published under the copyright owner's authority before January 1, 1978, without a proper copyright notice, all copyright protection for that work was permanently lost in the United States. The new copyright law does not provide retroactive protection for those works.

Copyright Registration

In general, copyright registration is a legal formality intended to make a public record of the basic facts of a particular copyright. However, except in one specific situation*, registration is not a condition of copyright protection. Even though registration is not generally a requirement for protection, the copyright law provides several inducements or advantages to encourage copyright owners to make registration. Among these advantages are the following:

*Under sections 405 and 406 of the Copyright Act, copyright registration may be required to preserve a copyright that would otherwise be invalidated because of the omission of the copyright notice from the published copies or phonorecords, or omission of the name or date, or a certain error in the year date.

Registration establishes a public record of the copyright claim;

Registration is ordinarily necessary before any infringement suits may be filed in court;

If made before or within 5 years of publication, registration will establish prima facie evidence in court of the validity of the copyright and of the facts stated in the certificate; and

If registration is made within 3 months after publication of the work or prior to an infringement of the work, statutory damages and attorney's fees will be available to the copyright owner in court actions. Otherwise, only an award of actual damages and profits is available to the copyright owner.

Registration may be made at any time within the life of the copyright. Unlike the law before 1978, when a work has been registered in unpublished form, it is not necessary to make another registration when the work becomes published (although the copyright owner may register the published edition, if desired).

Registration Procedures

In General

If you choose to register your work, send the following three elements to the Copyright Office **in the same envelope or package**:

(1) A properly completed application form;
(2) A fee of $10 for each application;
(3) A deposit of the work being registered. The deposit requirements will vary in particular situations. The general requirements are as follows:

If the work is unpublished, one complete copy or phonorecord.

If the work was first published in the U.S. on or after January 1, 1978, two complete copies or phonorecords of the best edition.

If the work was first published in the U.S. before January 1, 1978, two complete copies or phonorecords of the work as first published.

If the work was first published outside the U.S., whenever published, one complete copy or phonorecord of the work as first published.

If the work is a contribution to a collective work, and published after January 1, 1978, one complete copy or phonorecord of the best edition of the collective work.

NOTE: COMPLETE THE APPLICATION FORM USING INK PEN OR TYPEWRITER. After registration is completed, the application form becomes a part of the official permanent records of the Copyright Office so the application forms must meet archival standards. Therefore, applications must be submitted only on forms printed and issued by the Copyright Office and should be completed legibly in dark ink or typewritten.

Unpublished Collections

A work may be registered in unpublished form as a "collection," with one application and one fee, under the following conditions:

The elements of the collection are assembled in an orderly form;

The combined elements bear a single title identifying the collection as a whole;

The copyright claimant in all the elements and in the collection as a whole is the same; and

All the elements are by the same author, or, if they are by different authors, at least one of the authors has contributed copyrightable authorship to each element.

Unpublished collections are indexed in the *Catalog of Copyright Entries* only under the collective titles.

Special Deposit Requirements

The Copyright Act gives the Register of Copyrights authority to issue regulations making adjustments in the statutory deposit requirements. These regulations as now issued require or permit, for particular classes, the deposit of identifying material instead of copies or phonorecords, the deposit of only one copy or phonorecord where two would normally be required, and in some cases material other than complete copies of the best edition. For example, the regulations ordinarily require deposit of identifying material, such as photographs or drawings, when the work being registered has been reproduced in three-dimensional copies.

If you are unsure of the proper deposit required for your work, write to the Copyright Office for that information and describe the work you wish to register.

NOTE: CATALOGING IN PUBLICATION DIVISION. The Copyright Office is operationally separate from the Cataloging in Publication (CIP) Division. Correspondence concerning registration and the required deposit copies of books must be addressed to the Register of Copyrights, Copyright Office, Washington, D.C. 20559. A book may be copyrighted but not necessarily cataloged and added to the Library's collections. For information concerning the CIP program or for obtaining a catalog card number contact the CIP Division, Library of Congress, Washington, D.C. 20540.

Corrections and Amplifications of Existing Registrations

To deal with cases in which information in the basic registration later turns out to be incorrect or incomplete, the law provides for "the filing of an application for supplementary registration, to correct an error in a copyright registration or to amplify the information given in a registration." The information in a supplementary registration augments but does not supersede that contained in the earlier registration. Note also that a supplementary registration is not a substitute for an original registration or for a renewal registration. Form CA is available from the Copyright Office for making a supplementary registration. For further information about supplementary registrations, write for Circular R8.

Mandatory Deposit for Works Published in the United States with Notice of Copyright

Although a copyright registration is not required, the Copyright Act establishes a mandatory deposit requirement for works published with notice of copyright in the United States (see definition of "publication"). In general, the owner of copyright, or the owner of the right of first publication in the work, has a legal obligation to deposit in the Copyright Office, within 3 months of publication in the United States, two copies (or, in the case of sound recordings, two phonorecords) for the use of the Library of Congress. Failure to make the deposit can give rise to fines and other penalties, but does not affect copyright protection.

The Copyright Office has issued regulations *exempting* certain categories of works *entirely* from the mandatory deposit requirements, and reducing the obligation for certain other categories.

Use of Mandatory Deposit to Satisfy Registration Requirements

With respect to works published in the United States, the Copyright Act contains a special provision under which a single deposit can be made to satisfy both the deposit requirements for the Library and the registration requirements. The provision requires that, in order to have this dual effect, the copies or phonorecords must be "accompanied by the prescribed application and fee" for registration.

How Long Copyright Protection Endures

Works Originally Copyrighted on or after January 1, 1978

A work that is created (fixed in tangible form for the first time) on or after January 1, 1978, is automatically protected from the moment of its creation, and is ordinarily given a term enduring for the author's life, plus an additional 50 years after the author's death. In the case of "a joint work prepared by two or more authors who did not work for hire," the term lasts for 50 years after the last surviving author's death. For works made for hire, and for anonymous and pseudonymous works (unless the author's identity is revealed in Copyright Office records), the duration of copyright will be 75 years from publication or 100 years from creation, whichever is shorter.

Works that were created before the new law came into effect, but had neither been published nor registered for copyright before January 1, 1978, have been automatically brought under the statute and are now given Federal copyright protection. The duration of copyright in these works will generally be computed in the same way as for new works: the life-plus-50 or 75/100-year terms will apply to them as well. However, all works in this category are guaranteed at least 25 years of statutory protection.

Works Copyrighted before January 1, 1978

Under the law in effect before 1978, copyright was secured either on the date a work was published, or on the date of registration if the work was registered in unpublished form. In either case, the copyright endured for a first term of 28 years from the date it was secured. During the last (28th)

year of the first term, the copyright was eligible for renewal. The new
copyright law has extended the renewal term from 28 to 47 years for
copyrights that were subsisting on January 1, 1978. However, the
copyright *must* be timely renewed to receive the 47-year period of added
protection. For more detailed information on the copyright term, write to
the Copyright Office and request Circulars R15a and R15t. For information
on how to search the Copyright Office records concerning the copyright
status of a work, ask for Circular R22.

Transfer of Copyright

Any or all of the exclusive rights, or any subdivision of those rights, of the
copyright owner may be transferred, but the transfer of *exclusive* rights is
not valid unless that transfer is in writing and signed by the owner of the
rights conveyed (or such owner's duly authorized agent). Transfer of a
right on a nonexclusive basis does not require a writing.

A copyright may also be conveyed by operation of law and may be
bequeathed by will or pass as personal property by the applicable laws of
intestate succession.

Copyright is a personal property right, and it is subject to the various
state laws and regulations that govern the ownership, inheritance, or
transfer of personal property as well as terms of contracts or conduct of
business. For information about relevant state laws consult an attorney.

Transfers of copyright are normally made by contract. The Copyright
Office does not have or supply any forms for such transfers. However, the
law does provide for the recordation in the Copyright Office of transfers of
copyright. Although recordation is not required to make a valid transfer as
between the parties, it does provide certain legal advantages and may be
required to validate the transfer as against third parties. For information on
recordation of transfers and other documents related to copyright, write to
the Copyright Office.

Termination of Transfers

Under the old law, the copyright in a work generally reverted to the
author, if living, or if the author was not living, to other specified
beneficiaries, provided a renewal claim was registered in the 28th year of
the original term. The new law drops the renewal feature except for works
already in their first term of statutory protection when the new law took
effect. Instead, the new law generally permits termination of the grant of
rights after 35 years under certain conditions by serving written notice on
the transferee within specified time limits.

For works already under statutory copyright protection, the new law provides a similar right of termination covering the newly added years that extended the former maximum term of the copyright from 56 to 75 years. For further information, write to the Copyright Office.

International Copyright Protection

There is no such thing as an "international copyright" that will automatically protect an author's writings throughout the entire world. Protection against unauthorized use in a particular country depends, basically, on the national laws of that country. However, most countries do offer protection to foreign works under certain conditions, and these conditions have been greatly simplified by international copyright treaties and conventions.

The United States is a member of the Universal Copyright Convention (the UCC), which came into force on September 16, 1955. Generally, a work by a national or domiciliary of a country that is a member of the UCC or a work first published in a UCC country may claim protection under the UCC. If the work bears the notice of copyright in the form and position specified by the UCC, this notice will satisfy and substitute for any other formal conditions a UCC member country would otherwise impose to secure copyright.

An author who wishes protection for his or her work in a particular country should first find out the extent of protection of foreign works in that country. If possible, this should be done before the work is published anywhere, since protection may often depend on the facts existing at the time of **first** publication.

If the country in which protection is sought is a party to one of the international copyright conventions, the work may generally be protected by complying with the conditions of the convention. Even if the work cannot be brought under an international convention, protection under the specific provisions of the country's national laws may still be possible. Some countries, however, offer little or no copyright protection for foreign works.

Who May File an Application Form

The following persons are legally entitled to submit an application form:

The author. This is either the person who actually created the work, or, if the work was made for hire, the employer or other person for whom the work was prepared.

The copyright claimant. The copyright claimant is defined in the Copyright Office regulations as either the author of the work or a person or organization that has obtained ownership of all of the rights under the copyright initially belonging to the author. This category includes a person or organization who has obtained by contract the right to claim legal title to the copyright in an application for copyright registration.

The owner of exclusive right(s). Under the new law, any of the exclusive rights that go to make up a copyright and any subdivision of them can be transferred and owned separately, even though the transfer may be limited in time or place of effect. The term "copyright owner" with respect to any one of the exclusive rights contained in a copyright refers to the owner of that particular right. Any owner of an exclusive right may apply for registration of a claim in the work.

The duly authorized agent of such author, other copyright claimant, or owner of exclusive right(s). Any person authorized to act on behalf of the author, other copyright claimant, or owner of exclusive right(s) may apply for registration.

There is no requirement that applications be prepared or filed by an attorney.

Applications Forms

For Original Registration
Form TX: for published and unpublished nondramatic literary works
Form PA: for published and unpublished works of the performing arts (musical and dramatic works, pantomimes and choreographic works, motion pictures, and other audiovisual works)
Form VA: for published and unpublished works of the visual arts (pictorial, graphic, and sculptural works)
Form SR: for published and unpublished sound recordings

For Renewal Registration
Form RE: for claims to renewal copyright in works copyrighted under the old law

For Corrections and Amplifications

Form CA: for supplementary registration to correct or amplify information given in the Copyright Office record of an earlier registration

Other Forms for Special Purposes

Form GR/CP: an adjunct application to be used for registration of a group of contributions to periodicals in addition to an application Form TX, PA, or Va

Form IS: request for issuance of an import statement under the manufacturing provisions of the Copyright Act.

For more detailed information about all these forms, write for Circular R1c.

Application forms are supplied by the Copyright Office free of charge. Photocopies of application forms are *not* acceptable for registration.

Mailing Instructions

All material and communications sent to the Copyright Office should be addressed to the Register of Copyrights, Library of Congress, Washington, D.C. 20559.

The application, deposit (copies or phonorecords), and fee should be mailed in the same package.

Index